SEROLOGICAL DIAGNOSTIX

Publication Number 655
AMERICAN LECTURE SERIES®

A Monograph in
The BANNERSTONE DIVISION *of*
AMERICAN LECTURES IN LIVING CHEMISTRY

Edited by
I. NEWTON KUGELMASS, M.D., Ph.D., Sc.D.
Consultant to the Departments of Health and Hospitals
New York, New York

SEROLOGICAL DIAGNOSTIX

By

LUCIO NUZZOLO, M.S., M.D., L.D.
Assistant, Istituto di Clinica
Medica Generale e Metodologia Clinica
Università di Roma
Rome, Italy

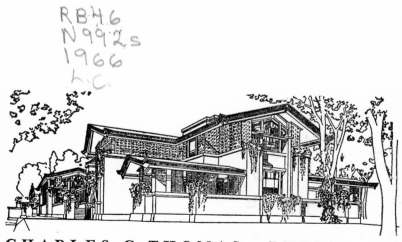

CHARLES C THOMAS · PUBLISHER
Springfield · Illinois · U.S.A.

Published and Distributed Throughout the World by
CHARLES C THOMAS • PUBLISHER
BANNERSTONE HOUSE
301-327 East Lawrence Avenue, Springfield, Illinois, U.S.A.
NATCHEZ PLANTATION HOUSE
735 North Atlantic Boulevard, Fort Lauderdale, Florida, U.S.A.

With THOMAS BOOKS *careful attention is given to all details of
manufacturing and design. It is the Publisher's desire to present books
that are satisfactory as to their physical qualities and artistic possibilities
and appropriate for their particular use.* THOMAS BOOKS *will be true
to those laws of quality that assure a good name and good will.*

Printed in the United States of America
P-4

This book is dedicated

to

PROFESSOR LUIGI CONDORELLI

and

DOCTOR JOHN C. SNYDER

FOREWORD

Our Living Chemistry Series was conceived by Editor and Publisher to advance the newer knowledge of chemical medicine in the cause of clinical practice. The interdependence of chemistry and medicine is so great that physicians are turning to chemistry, and chemists to medicine in order to understand the underlying basis of life processes in health and disease. Once chemical truths, proofs, and convictions become sound foundations for clinical phenomena, key hybrid investigators clarify the bewildering panorama of biochemical progress for application in everyday practice, stimulation of experimental research, and extension of postgraduate instruction. Each of our monographs thus unravels the chemical mechanisms and clinical management of many diseases that have remained relatively static in the minds of medical men for three thousand years. Our new Series is charged with the *nisus élan* of chemical wisdom, supreme in choice of international authors, optimal in standards of chemical scholarship, provocative in imagination for experimental research, comprehensive in discussions of scientific medicine, and authoritative in chemical perspective of human disorders.

Dr. Nuzzolo of Rome presents the laboratory procedures by which foreign materials, antigens, and antibodies may be measured qualitatively and quantitatively for the diagnosis of bacterial, parasitic, mycotic, viral, and rickettsial infections, followed by decisive tests of the blood and blood-forming organs indispensable in the diagnosis of hematologic and systemic diseases. Without neglecting the methods of investigation which are still in the realm of research, the author stresses those proven effective in current practice with critical interpretations while indicating difficulties, uncertainties, and sources of error. The practitioner is thus informed of three things about every laboratory procedure: when to use it, how to interpret the results, what limitations affect the interpretation in the skillful blending of the history and physical examination. When a difficult clinical problem is encountered or the use of involved techniques is necessary, it is well for the clinician and pathologist to exchange views to evolve a course of action for optimal data and for optimal management with minimal laboratory tests. Elaborate procedures play an important part in medicine today, but I sometimes wonder if we are not inclined to forget that the most important instrument in clinical diagnosis must always be the trained mind of the alert clinician.

The science of serology emerged before the turn of the century from discoveries of humoral immunity. Charrin (1889) observed that the cells of B. pyocyaneus clumped in immune serum; Durham (1896), the clumping specific for each bacterium; Widal (1897), the specific agglutination in the diagnosis of typhoid. Bordet (1898) also produced specific agglutinins by injecting animals with erythrocytes, thereby enabling Landsteiner (1900) to classify human blood groups. Bordet (1901) then worked out the complement-fixation test which Wassermann (1906) applied to the serodiagnosis of syphilis. Nuttal (1903) used the newly discovered precipitation reaction for the serologic identification of blood stains and the analysis of immune processes. Koch's (1890) discovery of the tuberculin reaction led to Ricket's (1902) observation of anaphylaxis, von Pirquet's (1905) description of serum disease, and the Prausnitz-Küstner (1921) reaction. Ehrlich (1908) advanced the chemical theory to account for all the immunologic phenomena, while Landsteiner (1944) discovered immunologic specificity in the study of microbial agents of disease.

Infectious diseases are produced by living agents, viruses, rickettsial, bacteria, fungi, protozoa, or nematodes. Confirmation of a presumptive diagnosis depends upon laboratory procedures involving direct demonstration of the causative organism, or proof of its presence by indirect means. Diagnostic procedures are not absolute, hence the dire need for careful interpretation of laboratory data. The presence of the specific organism is not the only factor of infection, nor is the isolation of bacteria from the body the whole of diagnosis. The most virulent of human bacteria are still capable of maintaining a harmless existence in the tissues: The buccal cavity may harbor the pneumococcus, the hemolytic streptococcus, the corynebacterium diphtheriae; the gallbladder, the typhoid bacillus; the renal pelvis, the colon bacillus—without affecting the host. A throat culture containing beta-hemolytic streptococci does not rule out diphtheria; a nasal culture containing staphylococci does not indicate staphylococcal sinusitis in a patient with headaches; a positive serologic test for syphilis may forewarn incipient lupus erythematosus; a positive candida albicans stool culture does not confirm intestinal moniliasis.

Blood diseases affect the red blood corpuscles, leucocytes, platelets, clotting components, and cells of the reticuloendothelial system, hence hematologic diagnosis is determined by accurate blood counts and morphological studies of the cells in peripheral blood and bone marrow. A blood film reveals more from qualitative perspective than from quantitative counting. A coup d'oeil unravels unsuspected abnormality of erythrocytes or absence of platelets while enumeration merely yields relative figures. A bone marrow aspiration or trephine biopsy adds to the basic morphologic data, but precise diagnosis requires further biochemical, physiologic, or immunologic determinations. Quantitative studies of erythrocyte disorders will be rewarded by measuring serum iron and saturation of the iron-binding protein, plasma vitamin B_{12}, total circulating red blood cell mass, rate of blood cell destruction, Coombs' test, plasma-free hemoglobin content; osmotic fragility, hemoglobin electrophoretic pattern, erythrocyte sickling, red-cell glucose-6-phosphate dehydrogenase content. Quantitative studies of leucocyte disorders are fewer and less dependable, though equally important, in establishing the final diagnosis. However, quantitative studies of blood-clotting disorders have come into their own, enabling greater precision in the differential diagnosis of enzyme and platelet deviations. It is the modest, not the presumptuous inquirer who makes real advances in the discovery of clinical truths, at the bedside and in the laboratory. Medical progress depends upon how, not upon where, the work is done, for clinical science emerges from the intelligence, imagination, and insight of the investigator, whether his data derives from molecules or man and clinical wisdom from the knowledge, experience, and understanding of the clinician.

I. NEWTON KUGELMASS, M.D., PH.D., SC.D., *Editor*

PREFACE

THE CONTINUOUS EVOLUTION in the field of diagnostic serology offered several ways for planning a book on this subject. To determine which one to follow, the subject was discussed with various people involved in routine serological work. Among these were doctors, students and laboratory personnel. In other words, we consulted people of different levels having a sufficient background to understand and discuss the matter.

The final decision was to avoid a necessarily short, and thus mediocre, introduction to immunity and immunology, considering also the fact that excellent, up-to-date literature is easily available. We decided to get right into the subject, trying to give a number of experimented and reliable techniques, with the addition of some notes, aimed to help in the practical application of them. Some of the techniques described herein are classical while others are rather new.

The fields of bacteriology, mycology, parasitology, virology and hematology, from an immunological standpoint, are included. This does not mean that every existing technique is mentioned in the book. We tried to select what we thought to be most profitable for a medium-sized laboratory or for practitioners and students facing unusual problems. We hope that the bibliographic references will help in understanding better whatever may be inadequate in our work.

CONTENTS

Contents

SEROLOGICAL DIAGNOSTIX

I

SEROLOGICAL DIAGNOSTIX IN BACTERIAL DISEASES

1. BACILLUS ANTHRACIS (Malignant Pustule)

For postmortem diagnosis of B. anthracis infection perform a

Precipitin Test (Ascoli Test) [13]

Boil 1.0 to 2.0 gm of spleen from an animal which has presumably
   died of anthrax in 10.0 to 12.0 ml of saline. Prepare controls
   from normal spleen and from some animals infected with
   B. anthracis, using the same method.
Filter the extracts through filter-paper.
Distribute 1 to 1.5 ml of specific precipitating serum in three
   serology tubes, and an equal amount of normal serum in two
   tubes.
Carefully form 1 to 1.5 ml layers of spleen extracts.

Schematically:

Tubes n°	1	2	3	4	5
Tissue extracts	unknown spleen	normal spleen	infected spleen	infected spleen	unknown spleen
Precipitating sera	*	*	*		
Normal sera				*	*

When test is positive, a ring of precipitate will develop in tubes
1 and 3.

   Agglutination tests in B. anthracis infections are not reliable
due to the instability of the antigen suspensions.

2. BACTEROIDES [31]

   Serological tests for Bacteroides infections are not normally
used. Significant values for the most common of these agents are
as follows:

B. ramosus (Ramibacterium ramosum): The patient's sera may agglutinate to a dilution of up to $\frac{1}{100}$ the homologous strain.

B. funduliformis (Spherosphorus funduliformis): * Agglutination may be observed up to dilutions of $\frac{1}{800}$.

B. fragilis (Ristella fragilis): Sera do not agglutinate homologous strains.

3. BRUCELLA (Brucellosis)

Agglutinins, in Brucella infections, appear in the patient's sera eight to ten days after the onset of the disease.

Agglutination Test (Wright Test) [1, 25]

Preparation of the antigen [20]

B. melitensis, abortus and suis are very similar antigenically. Any one of the three types can be used in preparing antigen with satisfactory results. B. abortus, however, is considered the best choice.

Some strains of B. abortus are particularly suitable for laboratory work, both for their antigenicity and for the fact that they are avirulent.

Inoculate slants of infusion or trypticase soy agar with a small amount of a 48 hr broth culture of Brucella.

Incubate at 37° C for 48 hr.

Wash the bacterial growth as described on page 19; the physiological saline (ps) should be formolized or phenolized to 0.5 per cent.

Store the suspension at 4° C for 48 hr, perform a sterility test and, if the result is negative, store the stock suspension at 4° C. For best results, renew the stock every ten days.

When used, dilute the stock suspension to a concentration comparable to tube N°3 of the McFarland nephelometer.†

Technique of the test

Follow the technique described on page 19.‡

Incubate at 37° C for about 15 hr, then for 12 hr at room temperature.

---

* In B. funduliformis infections, after about ten days from the onset of the disease, a *flocculation test* can be performed, using equal parts of patient's serum and a mixture containing 14 parts of an alcoholic extract of the antigen and

Interpretation of the results

A titer of $\frac{1}{80}$ is considered significant. An increase of titers, in the course of the disease, is also considered significant for diagnosis.

Coombs Test in Brucellosis [26]

In some brucellosis cases the agglutination test may be negative because of the presence of incomplete antibodies which inhibit reactions of specific antibodies. A Coombs test is then necessary.

Technique of the test

First part.

Perform an agglutination test as described above.

Second part.

Centrifuge negative tubes at 3,000 rpm for 45 min.

Discard supernatant.

Add 2.0 to 3.0 ml of ps and centrifuge again.

Discard the supernatant and repeat washing and centrifuging twice.

1 part of Sumatra benzoin tincture; after incubation at 37° C for 4 to 12 hr, flocculation can be observed in positive sera.

† McFARLAND SCALE [11]

Tube n°		BaCl₂ 1%	H₂ SO₄ 1%	Cells x 10⁶
1	ml	0.1	9.9	300
2	ml	0.2	9.8	600
3	ml	0.3	9.7	900
4	ml	0.4	9.6	1200
5	ml	0.5	9.5	1500
6	ml	0.6	9.4	1800
7	ml	0.7	9.3	2100
8	ml	0.8	9.2	2400
9	ml	0.9	9.1	2700
10	ml	1.0	9.0	3000

‡ In brucellosis agglutination test, a specific conglutination may sometimes be observed both with normal sera or those from different diseases. On occasion "prozone" phenomenon may also be observed. It is convenient, therefore, to heat the sera at 56° C for 30 min in order to destroy conglutinins. The use of high dilutions will prevent erroneous interpretations when zone phenomena are observed; the use of hypertonic solutions (NaCl 5 per cent) in sera dilutions will also prevent zone phenomena. Antigens should be stored for rather short periods.[25]

Shake the sediment and add one drop of human antiglobulin
serum, previously absorbed on Brucella antigen, to each tube.
Incubate at 37° C for 13 hr.

Read for results.

The titer of agglutination is the highest dilution of serum in
which agglutination is observed.

4. CLOSTRIDIUM BOTULINUM

No agglutination or complement-fixation reactions are reliable for diagnostic purposes.

5. ERISIPELOTHRIX RHUSIOPATHIAE[29] (Erysipeloid)
(Bacillus Erysipelatus Suis)

Immunologic reactions are seldom used for the diagnosis of
E. rhusiopathiae infections because of the weak and short antibodies response in human beings.

Titers over $\frac{1}{85}$ are considered significant in agglutination
tests.

Complement-fixation tests are not reliable.

6. HEMOPHILUS DUCREYI (Chancroid)

The agglutination test is used as an aid in H. ducreyi infections.

Agglutination Test[6, 22]

Preparation of the antigen

Cultivate H. ducreyi on D'Antona-Valensin (DV) medium at 36
to 37° C for three or four days.

Wash the surface growth with buffer saline (pH 7 to 7.2).

Add formol to the suspension to a concentration of 0.2 per cent.

Incubate at 37° C for two to four days.

Make a sterility test in DV medium and in thyoglicollate.

If sterile, the suspension is ready for use.

Technique of the test

For the dilution of serum and technique of the test, follow
the table on page 20.

Interpretation of the results

Visible agglutination is observed with positive sera.

7. HEMOPHILUS PERTUSSIS (Pertussis)

The agglutination test is usually positive several days after the onset of the disease or during convalescence, thus being of little help for an early diagnosis. The same occurs with the complement-fixation test, which is not widely used.

Agglutination Test [2, 14]

Preparation of the antigen

Wash 48 hr old H. pertussis cultures on glycerin-potato blood agar with ps.
Suspend organisms homogeneously in sodium citrate solution 3.8 per cent and standardize against strong, weakly positive and negative agglutinating antisera as follows:

> Dilute bacillary suspension to a concentration comparable to tube N° 4 of McFarland nephelometer;
> Mix 0.1 ml of antiserum to 0.1 ml of diluted antigen;
> Mix 0.1 ml of saline to 0.1 ml of diluted antigen, for control of autoagglutination;
> Shake for 3 min, and
> Add 0.5 ml of saline to all tubes.
> Only strong agglutination is considered positive.

Add methylene blue to a satisfactory concentration obtained through repeated tests with positive antisera.
Add Merthiolate to $1/10,000$ concentration.
Distribute about $1/40$ ml in capillary tubes to use separately in single tests or in small dropper bottles.
Store at 4° C.

Serum

Either serum or single drops of blood from finger or ear, obtained as for blood count, can be tested.

Technique of the test

Place one drop of the blue antigen on a 7.5 cm x 2.5 cm rec-
    tangular piece of cardboard or hard paper, reddish for blood,
    white for serum.
Spread the drop of the blue antigen with a thin glass rod to cover
    the surface of about ½ in diameter circle.
Add an equal volume of serum or blood to the antigen.
Prepare two controls, with known positive antiserum, for activity
    of the antigen, and with saline, for autoagglutination of the
    antigen.
Stir the mixture a few seconds and then gently shake the paper
    horizontally for 1 min.
Read the results.

Interpretation of the results

A visible agglutination, stained blue, is visible with positive
sera.

8. LEPTOSPIRA [32] (Leptospirosis)

Several tests are used in the diagnosis of leptospirosis, but the
agglutination test is preferred.

Agglutination Test (Martin and Pettit Test) [10]

The agglutination test can be performed in many different
ways. The use of living and highly virulent antigens is recommended for its specificity. The microscopic method, on dark-field
observation, is the one of choice.

In macroscopic agglutination tests, formolized antigens are
used.

Dilute the serum to be tested logarithmically, in saline, begin-
    ning from $\frac{1}{10}$.
Mix 0.1 ml of each dilution, separately, with 0.9 ml of a seven to
    nine days growth of leptospirae suspension: the first final
    dilution will now be equal to 10^{-2}.
Incubate at 37° C for 2 hr.
Place one loopful of each serum dilution-antigen suspension mix-
    ture on a slide for dark-field observation.

Interpretation of the results

The final readings are not evaluated in the same way by all researchers. Some consider the titer of the serum as given by the highest dilution in which agglutination is observed. Some others take as a final titer the serum dilution by which the 50 per cent of organisms are agglutinated.

A titer of $\frac{1}{100}$ and over is of diagnostic importance.

Absorption of the agglutinins [21] (Castellani, Schuffner-Bohlander test)

When cross agglutinations among various strains of leptospira are observed, the following technique for the absorption of the agglutinins is employed. For the principles of the method, see page 21.

Add 0.5 ml of formalin to 100.0 ml of a rich Leptospira suspension.
Centrifuge at 10,000 rpm for 20 min.
Dilute serum to be tested $\frac{1}{3,000}$.
Mix 1 volume of the diluted serum with 9 volumes of Leptospira sediment.
Keep at room temperature for 24 hr.
Centrifuge at 10,000 rpm for 5 min.
Recuperate the supernatant and use it for the standard agglutination test.

The tests of complement-fixation, precipitation, flocculation, coagulation, protection, etc. are not commonly used because of their rather poor specificity.

However, the complement-fixation test has given, in some instances, good results. Many methods for the preparation of the antigens have been employed.

9. LISTERIA MONOCYTOGENES

In L. monocytogenes infections, serological tests are not yet widely used for various reasons. Sera from apparently healthy individuals, with no history of such infection, may give positive responses by agglutination, and sometimes high titers may be reached.

Some strains of Streptococcus fecalis have serological relationships with L. monocytogenes of the serotypes I, II, and III.

Besides the agglutination test, a complement-fixation test has been used with uncertain results: a significant titer would be $\frac{1}{10}$.

Antigen-fixation Test [12]

This test has been recently and successfully experimented on a number of sera having antibodies to L. monocytogenes. The procedure used in the experiments will be described as a standard method.

Preparation of the antigen

The L. monocytogenes strain used is n° 3-54, serotype IVb.

Maintain the strain in tryptose agar (Difco) at 4° C and periodically pass it in mice for preservation of virulence and of antigenic properties.

Cultivate a bulk of cells, freshly reisolated from mice, in a brain-heart infusion broth at 30° C on a mechanical shaker for 48 hr.

Inactivate, adding formalin to a 0.6 per cent concentration.

Centrifuge at 4,400 rpm for 90 min.

Resuspend the sediment in distilled H_2O, employing 5.0 ml of diluent to 1.0 of cells.

Staining procedure

Filter a solution of Delafield's hematoxylin, modified according to Harris (Nat. Anilin Chemical Co.), and add 1.0 ml of the solution to 5.0 ml of the bacterial suspension.

Incubate at room temperature for 24 hr.

Wash and centrifuge three times the stained cells with phosphate buffered saline (pbs) at pH 7.0—the last centrifugation to be carried at 4,400 rpm for 90 min in a graduated tube.

Determine the volume of the packed cells.

Add rabbit serum to the cells at a ratio of 3.0 ml to 1.0 ml of cells; the serum should be previously absorbed with Lysteria cells and diluted to 50 per cent with pbs.

Add merthiolate to a final concentration of $\frac{1}{10,000}$; store at 4° C for a maximum of one week.

Technique of the test

Use a standard 4 mm loop for placing the stained antigen on strips
of ED 609 filter paper (Eaton-Dikeman Co., Mount Holly
Springs, Penn.).

Wash the loop in saline and flame.

Using the same loop, place the undiluted serum to be tested on
the antigen, covering it completely.

Soak the paper strip in pbs (pH 7.0) until the level of it is about
½ in below the antigen-serum area.

The saline will rise to the top of the filter paper by capillarity.

Interpretation of the results

With specific antiserum, the stained antigen remains firmly at-
tached to the filter paper at the point of its application. With
sera containing "cross-reacting" antibodies, the stain fades towards the top of the strip.

In control strips, where antigen has been overlaid with saline
and normal serum, the stained antigen moves towards the top
of the strip.

10. MALLEOMYCES MALLEI (Glanders)

Agglutination and complement-fixation tests are used in the
diagnosis of glanders. A C-F test, though slower in reaching
positivity, is more specific than the agglutination test and may
reach titers as high as $\frac{1}{640}$.

Agglutination Test (Povitsky Test)

Preparation of the antigen [5]

1°.

Wash a 48 hr M. mallei growth on glycerin-potato-veal agar with
a small amount of ps.

Transfer the suspension to a new tube.

Heat at 70° C for 1 hr.

Store at 4° C for up to two months.

Dilute in ps to a faint opalescence before use.

or

2°. [3]

Incubate beef extract-glycerol agar plates, heavily seeded with
    M. mallei, at 37° C for 24 hr.
Harvest the growth with 0.5 per cent phenolized saline and
    homogenize with glass beads,
Incubate at 37 °C for two to four days.
Perform a sterility test, if negative.
Filter through sterilized filter paper.
Dilute to a concentration comparable to tube N° 3 of McFarland
    nephelometer before using.

Technique of the test

Dilute 0.1 ml of serum in 3.9 ml of ps to obtain a dilution of $\frac{1}{40}$.
Distribute 3.0 ml of the antigen to each of five tubes.
Add 0.1 ml of the $\frac{1}{40}$ serum dilution to the first tube, thus ob-
    taining a $\frac{1}{1,200}$ dilution.
Add 0.075 ml of the $\frac{1}{40}$ serum dilution to the second tube; final
    dilution $\frac{1}{1,600}$.
Add 0.06 ml of the $\frac{1}{40}$ serum dilution to the third tube; final dilu-
    tion $\frac{1}{2,000}$.
Add 0.1 ml of known positive antiserum to the fourth tube for
    antigen activity control and reference titer.
Add 0.1 ml of known negative serum to the fifth tube for speci-
    ficity of the antigen and autoagglutination control.
Shake well and incubate at 37° C for 2 hr.
(Positive reactions may appear within 1 hr.)
Place at 4° C for about 12 hr.
Read for results.

Interpretation of the results

When the test is positive, the upper part of the liquid is clear
and an irregular sediment settles at the bottom of the tube. If
the test is negative, the upper part of the liquid is cloudy and a
sharp sedimentation forms at the bottom of the tube.

Control tubes 4 and 5 should be respectively positive and
negative.

Titers over $\frac{1}{320}$ and increase in titers are of diagnostic value;
titers may reach $\frac{1}{2,560}$.

Complement-fixation Test

Preparation of the antigen

Cultivate organisms as described in 1° for the preparation of agglutinating antigen.

Wash surface growth with formolized saline 0.5 per cent.

Incubate at 37° C for four days.

Make a sterility test.

Centrifuge at 5 to 6,000 rpm.

Recuperate the supernatant and add Merthiolate to $\frac{1}{5,000}$ concentration.

Store at 4° C.

11. MALLEOMYCES PSEUDOMALLEI [5] (Melioidosis)

Agglutination and complement-fixation tests are used. Cross-reactions are observed in both tests with M. mallei. Titers are generally higher for the homologous antigen. For the preparation of M. pseudomallei antigen for the agglutination test, the same method described in 2° for M. mallei can be used, with formolized saline (0.1 per cent) to preserve flagellar antigens.

12. MYCOBACTERIUM LEPRAE (Leprosy)

Many serological tests for the diagnosis of leprosy have been experimented; however, none have shown reliability because of the low sensitivity of the antigens and the poor specificity of the tests.

13. MYCOBACTERIUM TUBERCULOSIS (Tuberculosis)

Some serological tests are used as aids in the diagnosis of tuberculosis infections.[30]

Complement-fixation Test

This test is not used routinely due to the frequent cross-reactions observed in the course of other diseases such as cancer, syphilis, and malaria. In addition, the complement-fixing antibodies' response is usually poor.

The antigens for the test are commercially available and the technique is similar to the one used for the diagnosis of syphilis.

Agglutination Test (Arloing-Courmont Test)

This test is not commonly used.

Two-fold dilutions of the serum to be tested are challenged with a suspension of living organisms, well separated from each other.

A positive result ranges from $\frac{1}{10}$ to $\frac{1}{100}$ in adults; from $\frac{1}{5}$ in children, which indicates a recent infection. Sometimes the test is positive in typhoid infections.

Emoagglutination Test (Middlebrook and Dubost Test)

Sera from patients affected with some forms of tuberculosis infection often agglutinate sheep erythrocytes sensitized with tubercular antigens.

Components of the test:

(a) M. tuberculosis strain:

Cultivate a human strain of M. tuberculosis in Sauton medium at 37° C for thirty days.

Filter on filter paper.

Wash the bacilli on the filter, first with sterile distilled H_2O, and then with acetone.

Place the bacillary bulk in a Petri dish and let it dry at room temperature.

Suspend 3 gm of bacilli in 170.0 ml of phenol solution (88 per cent) and incubate at 35° C for 20 min.

Centrifuge at 3,000 rpm for 10 min and discard the supernatant.

Resuspend the sediment in phenol solution; incubate, centrifuge, and resuspend in phenol solution two more times.

Centrifuge and suspend the sediment in acetone twice.

Centrifuge again and discard the supernated acetone.

Let the bacilli dry at room temperature.

Grind the bacilli in a mortar.

0.5 gm of the ground bacilli are mixed with 65.0 ml of isotonic H_2O solution (NaCl 0.55 per cent; Na_2HPO_4 0.50 per cent; methyl alcohol 20 per cent).

Incubate the suspension at 35° C for 20 hr with frequent shaking.
Centrifuge at 3,000 for 20 min.
Dialyze the supernatant with tap water for 6 hr and then for two
    days with distilled H_2O.
Concentrate the extract with a fan until it reaches the volume
    of 20.0 ml.
Bring to pH 7.0.
Add 0.52 ml of NaCl saturated solution.
Store at 4° C until used.

(b) Sheep erythrocytes:

Centrifuge 10.0 ml of sheep defibrinated blood in a graduated
    tube at 3,000 rpm for 10 min.
Discard supernatant and add to the sediment a volume of ps
    equal to six times the original volume.
Centrifuge at 3,000 rpm for 10 min.
Discard the supernatant and repeat the washing and centrifuging
    procedure five more times.

(c) Serum:

Dilute one-half of the serum to be tested with ps and inactivate
    at 56° C for 30 min.
Add 0.2 ml of washed, packed sheep erythrocytes to 2.0 ml of
    diluted, inactivated serum, and keep at room temperature
    for 20 min.
Centrifuge and repeat absorption on sheep erythrocytes to elimi-
    nate antisheep emoagglutinins possibly present in the serum.

Sheep erythrocytes sensitization

Suspend 0.5 ml of packed erythrocytes in 10.0 ml of the bacilli
    extract.
Incubate in water bath at 37° C for 2 hr, shaking frequently.
Centrifuge and wash in ps three times.
Resuspend the last sediment in 95.5 ml of ps.

Technique of the test

Prepare a serial two-fold dilution of serum beginning from ½
    and up to $\frac{1}{256}$.

Distribute 0.4 ml of serum dilutions in two sets of serology tubes.

Add 0.4 ml of sensitized sheep erythrocytes at a 0.5 per cent concentration in ps, to the first set of tubes, and the same amount of unsensitized sheep erythrocytes, at the same concentration, to the second set as controls for possible spontaneous agglutination.

Shake well the whole and incubate at 37° C for 2 hr.

Perform the first reading; the definitive one is made after 10 hr of incubation.

Interpretation of the results

When the test is positive, a granular sedimentation will be observed. Under gentle shaking a granular suspension will appear.

A significant titer starts from ⅛ to 1/16.

Agglutination is often positive in caseous pneumonia, but rarely in other types of tuberculosis lesions.

Positive agglutination may be observed in leprosy.

Note: A simpler method to sensitize sheep erythrocytes can be applied as follows:

Dilute four times normal strength tuberculin (Lederle Labs, Pearl River, NY) with 2 volumes of phosphate-buffered saline (pbs).

Mix forty-eight volumes of such dilution to one volume of washed, sedimented sheep erythrocytes.

Incubate at 37° C for 2 hr, shaking frequently.

Centrifuge at 3,000 rpm for 10 min and discard the supernatant.

Wash and centrifuge three more times in pbs.

Resuspend the washed sensitized sheep erythrocytes in pbs to a 0.5 per cent concentration.

Store at 4° C and use within three days. Discard if hemolysis appears.

14. PASTEURELLA TULARENSIS (Tularemia)

Agglutinating antibodies appear about ten days after the onset of the disease.

Agglutination Test

Preparation of the antigen[20]

In preparing P. tularensis antigens, the use of nonvirulent strains (i.e., P. tularensis B-38 strain; National Institute of Health, Washington, D.C.) is recommended.

Wash off a 24 hr growth of P. tularensis on cystine blood agar at 37° C, using 2.0 ml of sterile ps.

Inoculate two loopfuls of the suspension in a new cystine blood agar slant.

Incubate at 37° C for 24 hr.

Wash off the growth with 0.5 per cent formolized sterile ps.

Repeat washing procedure three more times; store at 4° C.

Test for sterility on a suitable medium.

Dilute, when used, to a concentration comparable to tube N° 3 of the McFarland nephelometer.

Technique of the test

For dilution of sera and distribution of components of the test, see page 20.

Incubate at 37° C for 24 hr.

Read for results.

Interpretation of the results

A titer of $\frac{1}{200}$ and over is considered significant. Titers generally increase from the fourth to the seventh week, with a peak of $\frac{1}{1,280}$, $\frac{1}{2,560}$; the decrease starts on the eighth week.

An increase of the antibodies titer in the course of the disease has great diagnostic value.

In some cases of brucella infections, a cross-reaction with P. tularensis may occur. Under such conditions, an agglutinins saturation test will be performed. (See page 21.)

15. SALMONELLA [9, 19, 23, 27] (Typhoid, Paratyphoid Fever)

The main salmonella antigens are the somatic O and the flagellar H antigens. Some types (S. typhosa, hirschfeldi, ballerup, schottmuelleri, etc.) possess a somatic Vi (or virulence) antigen which, being at the periphery of the cell, prevents contact between the anti-O agglutinins and their specific somatic antigens, and thus agglutination.

Depending on the quantity of Vi antigens, salmonella possessing O antigens also can be agglutinated either by the anti-Vi serum, by the anti-O, or by both together. O and H antigens are formed by components having specific antigenic activity. O antigen components are designated by Roman numerals; flagellar phase 1 antigens are indicated by letters and those of phase 2 by Arabic numerals.

Through antigenic studies it has been possible to identify over 220 types of salmonella. It is, however, doubtful whether some of these types, being closely related antigenically, are to be considered different types or just varieties of certain types. In salmonella, agglutination can be of the somatic or of the flagellar type, according to the antigen acting in the reaction. The somatic type of agglutination is generally slow and the agglutinate is delicate and hardly dissociable by shaking; the flagellar type, on the contrary, is quick, the agglutinate being irregular and easily dissociable.

Agglutination Test (Widal Test)

This test is useful diagnostically when typhoid or paratyphoid infections are suspected. It reveals the presence, in the sera to be tested, of anti-H agglutinins, and positivity begins about ten days after the onset of the disease.

Preparation of H antigens

Either live or formolized organisms can be used as antigens, the latter being, naturally, much safer for laboratory workers.

(a) *Preparation of living antigens:*

Smooth and motile strains of S. typhi, paratyphi A, B, and C are used.

Transfer the strains on sterilized nutrient agar slants and incubate at 37° C for 18 hr.

Add 5.0 ml of sterile ps and wait for about 15 min, shake gently
and transfer the supernatant to another container.

Store the stock suspension at 4° C.

When used, dilute the suspension with sterile ps to bring it to
a concentration comparable to tube N° 3 of the McFarland
nephelometer.

(b) *Preparation of formolized antigens:*

Use the same media, strains, and incubation procedures described
above.

Wash the bacterial growth with 10.0 ml of sterile ps, formolized
0.5 per cent.

Centrifuge at 2,500 rpm for 10 min.

Discard the supernatant and add 10.0 ml of ps formolized 0.5
per cent.

Centrifuge.

Repeat such washing procedure two more times.

Store the suspension at 4° C for 48 hr.

Make a sterility test and, if negative, store at 4° C, ready for use.

When used, the same dilution of living antigens is prepared.

Technique of the test

Prepare a two-fold dilution of serum to be tested, beginning from
$\frac{1}{10}$ to $\frac{1}{640}$.

Distribute 1.0 ml of serum dilutions in separate tubes.

Add 1.0 ml of antigen to each tube: the final serum dilutions
range now from $\frac{1}{20}$ to $\frac{1}{1280}$.

The following controls are prepared:

      (a) one tube containing 1.0 ml of diluent to replace serum
for *autoagglutination control*, and

      (b) one tube containing 1.0 ml of known positive serum
for *antigen activity control*.

Shake well and incubate in water bath at 37° C for 12 to 18 hr.

Read for results.

Interpretation of the results

If the agglutination test is positive, a clearing up of the suspension will be observed and the cells will settle in a large, irregular area at the bottom of the tube, sometimes extending up the insides of the walls. A gentle shake will reveal medium-sized granules in the suspension.

If the test is negative, the cells will settle in a small round disc with sharp edges.

A salmonella agglutination test is considered significant when positivity is at least equal to $1/80$ for S. typhi and $1/160$ for S. paratyphi.

In sera obtained from vaccinated patients, titers should reach $1/320$ in a period of three months.

It is always useful, when the positivity is under the mentioned values, to repeat the test after some days.

AGGLUTINATION TEST CHART FOR TWO-FOLD DILUTIONS OF SERUM

Tubes n°	1	2	3	4	5	6	7	C_1	C_2
serum ml	0.2	transfer							known positive serum (1/20) 1.0 ml
ps ml	1.8	1.0	1.0	1.0	1.0	1.0	1.0 discard 1.0 ml	1.0	
serum dilution	1/10	20	40	80	160	320	640		
antigen ml	1.0	1.0	1.0	1.0	1.0	1.0	1.0	1.0	1.0
final serum dilution	1/20	40	80	160	320	640	1280		

Technique of the microscopic test

This test permits a quick answer using a living salmonella antigen prepared as described above.

Mix one drop of the serum to be tested with one drop of the antigen on a slide. (The serum can also be distributed in volumes of 0.8, 0.04, 0.02, 0.01 for more accurate titration.

Keep at room temperature for 20 min.

Cover with a cover-slide.

Observe under a microscope with a 6 to 8 lens.

Interpretation of the results

If the test is positive, it will be observed that the salmonella loose their motility and that 4 to 5 organisms will join together.

Saturation of the agglutinins

It may occur that a given serum agglutinates S. typhosa and paratyphosa antigens at the same time. This can be due either to a double infection or to a cross-reaction from common somatic antigen components.

In the latter case it is useful to recur to the agglutinin-saturation test. This because on confronting a serum with an antigen homologous to the "main" agglutinins both the main and the "minor" agglutinins disappear. On the contrary, if the minor antigen is used, only the minor agglutinins disappear.

Technique of the test

Assuming that a given serum agglutinates both S. typhi and paratyphi B:

Distribute 2.0 ml of serum in tubes I° and II°.
Add five loopfuls of bacteria grown on agar slants: S. typhi in tube I° and S. paratyphi in tube II°.
Incubate at 37° C for 2 hr.
Centrifuge at 2,000 rpm.
Recuperate sera I° and II°.
Repeat the agglutination test with S. typhi and paratyphi B respectively.

Interpretation of the results

(a) If serum I° does not agglutinate S. typhi and paratyphi B anymore, the main agglutinins were homologous to S. typhi and thus a typhoid infection can be suspected.

(b) If serum II° does not agglutinate S. typhi and paratyphi B, the main agglutinins were homologous to S. paratyphi B, and thus a paratyphoid infection can be suspected.

Schematically:

Tubes n°	I°	II°
Serum ml	2.0	2.0
S. typhi	+	
S. paratyphi B		+

Results after saturation:

Serum I° = NO agglutination for S. typhi and paratyphi
            B = main agglutinins S. typhi
Serum II° = NO agglutination for S. paratyphi B and
            typhi = main agglutinins S. paratyphi B.

Qualitative Agglutination Test

This method of agglutination reveals anti-O agglutinins and has the following advantages over the classical method previously described.

(a) Anti-O agglutinins appear earlier in the serum after an infection than do anti-H agglutinins.

(b) The disease can be, in some cases, caused by a strain of salmonella lacking H antigens.

(c) O antibody titer drops rapidly in vaccinated individuals and, in any case, seldom reaches significant values.

It is useful, however, to use both methods, employing O and H antigens in parallel.

Preparation of O antigens

There are two methods commonly used to prepare O antigens: one for nonmotile and one for motile strains.

(a) Preparation of antigen from nonmotile strains:

The technique is the same as that described for H antigens.

(b) Preparation of antigen from motile strains:

Prepare a thick suspension, washing off a motile strain of salmonella with sterile ps after 24 hr of incubation at 37° C.

Add an equal volume of absolute alcohol while stirring the suspension.

Incubate at 37° C for 24 hr.

Shake and leave at room temperature for 3 hr.

Add ½ volume of sterile ps in order to bring the alcohol concentration to 33 per cent.

When maintaining for long periods, store at 4° C.

The stock suspension is diluted in ps to a concentration comparable to tube N° 3 of the McFarland nephelometer.

Technique of the test at 37° C

The technique is the same as that previously described. The only difference is that for each serum two antigens, H and O, are used separately.

Incubate at 37° C for 2 hr.

Keep at room temperature for 10 min.

Read for final H antigen results.

Reincubate at 37° C and read again after 22 hr for O antigen results.

The different characteristics of the two types of agglutination have been described. (See page 18.)

Technique of the test at 52° C

The preparation for this test is similar to the one just described, the only difference being in the incubation phase.

Place the sets of tubes in a water bath at 52° C so that ⅓ of the serum-antigen mixture remains under the surface.

Incubate for 2 hr the set containing the H antigen and for 20 to 24 hr the one containing the O antigen.

After 10 min at room temperature read the results for the H antigen and after 1 hr for the O antigen.

Technique of the test after centrifugation

This technique is quick and reliable; many tubes, though, are to be centrifuged at the same time.

Prepare two separate dilutions of serum to be tested, $\frac{1}{10}$ and $\frac{1}{20}$.

Distribute components of the test as follows:

Tubes n°	1	2	3	4	5	6
Serum 1/10 ml	0.1	0.1				
Serum 1/20 ml			0.1	0.1		
H antigen ml		0.9		0.9		1.0
O antigen ml	0.9		0.9		1.0	
Final serum dilutions	1/100	1/100	1/200	1/200	contr.	contr.

Centrifuge at 3,000 rpm for 5 min.
Suspend the sediment in ps again and shake gently.
Read for results.

Interpretation of the results

If the suspension becomes homogeneous, the result is negative; if some agglutinates appear, the result is positive. Higher dilutions can be prepared.

Under such conditions, titers of 1/100 for S. typhi and paratyphi A (H and O), 1/200 for S. paratyphi B (H and O), and 1/400 for S. paratyphi C (H and O) can be considered significant.

In sera from vaccinated individuals, a titer over 1/100 in an O agglutination is significant for a salmonella infection.

If doubtful values should arise, repeated tests, simultaneously performed, showing a rise in the antibodies titer in the course of the disease will be meaningful in the diagnosis.

Vi Agglutination Test

Vi agglutinins appear in the serum of patients after about twelve days from the onset of the disease, etiologically caused by S. typhi and paratyphi having Vi antigens. The titer is low, generally around 1/25 and seldom reaching 1/50.

The antigen is prepared from S. typhi of the Vi Watson or Ty 68 strains.

The final dilutions of the sera commonly used are 1/10, 1/25, and 1/50.

An incubation period of 2 hr at 37° C is followed by a second one at room temperature lasting about 22 hr.

16. SHIGELLA [9, 19, 23, 28] (Bacillary Dysentery)

Agglutinins first appear in the patient's sera about ten days after the onest of the disease.

Agglutination Test

Agglutination with shigella antigens is of the O type. The antigens are prepared from strains of Sh. dysenteriae or flexneri, which are known to be free from heat-labile L antigens that may inhibit agglutination. The shigella antigenic picture is rather complicated. For this reason, cross-reactions and uncertain responses may often be observed. Thus serologic tests are not used routinely in shigellosis for diagnostic purposes.

Preparation of the antigen

Cultivate shigella strain on tryptose agar at 37° C for 48 hr.
Wash the bacterial growth with sterile bps (pH 7-7.2), formolized to 0.4 per cent.
Incubate at 37° C for two to four days.
Make a sterility test and, if negative,
Dilute with sterile bps to a concentration comparable to tube N° 3 of the McFarland nephelometer.

Technique of the test

For dilution of sera and distribution of the components see page 20.
Incubate at 37° C for 1 hr, then at room temperature for 23 hr.

Interpretation of the results

Agglutination is positive in about 70 per cent of the bacteriologically demonstrated cases. Cross-reactions between Sh. shiga and flexneri are common.

A titer is significant when it reaches values equal or superior to $\frac{1}{100}$ for the homologous antigen, and less than $\frac{1}{400}$ for the Sh. flexneri antigen in a Sh. shiga infection.

In a Sh. flexneri infection, titers are significant when equal or superior to $\frac{1}{400}$ for the homologous antigen and equal or less than $\frac{1}{50}$ for the Sh. shiga antigen.

17. SPIRILLUM MINUS (Sodoku)

Two tests can be performed for the following:

Serum spirocheticidal and spirochetilytic activity

A.

Mix one or two drops of serum taken from a convalescent of S. minus infection to the same amount of blood taken from a mouse experimentally infected with the same agent.

Microscopic examination will show, after a few minutes, the loss of motility by the microorganisms, followed by their disappearance.

B.

Inoculate a guinea pig intraperitoneally with a mixture of the convalescent's serum and spirilli, prepared as above.

In the peritoneal fluid, drawn every $\frac{1}{2}$ hr, no microorganisms are visible.

These tests can be positive up to twelve months after recovery.

Proteus OXK Agglutination Test (Weil-Felix test)

Very high agglutination titers have been observed with Proteus OXK antigens in rabbits infected with some strains of Sp. minus. Because of its aspecificity, this test is not commonly used in diagnostic serology.

Wassermann and Kahn Tests

The Wassermann and Kahn tests are irregularly positive or negative in the course of the disease, thus are not reliable in diagnostic serology.

18. STREPTOCOCCI

The titration of O-antistreptolysins is the method of choice in serological diagnosis of hemolytic streptococci infections.

O-antistreptolysins titration [7, 8, 15, 16, 17, 18, 22, 24]

Preparation of the materials for the test.

(a) Buffer solution (bs):

KH_2PO_4	1.4525	gm
$Na_2HPO_4 \cdot 2H_2O$	7.6006	gm
NaCl	4.8	gm
dist. H_2O	1.000	ml

(b) Rabbit erythrocytes:

Washed and centrifuged (2,000 rpm for 5 min) until the supernatant is clear, then suspended in bs to a concentration of 5 per cent.

(c) Serum:

Sterilely drawn and inactivated at 56° C for 30 min.

(d) O-streptolysin:

Commercially available. To be diluted in bs before use.

Technique of the test

Dilute serum in bs $\frac{1}{10}$, $\frac{1}{100}$, $\frac{1}{500}$ following the scheme:

serum	0.5 ml	transfer 1.0 ml	transfer 2.0 ml
bs	4.5 ml $\}\rightarrow$	9.0 ml $\}\rightarrow$	8.0 ml
dilutions of serum	$\frac{1}{10}$	$\frac{1}{100}$	$\frac{1}{500}$

Distribute the components in a set of twelve tubes according to the following scheme:
Prepare the following controls:

    (a) erythrocytes control for autohemolysis.
    (b) streptolysin control for hemolytic activity.

Shake well.
Incubate in water bath at 37° C for 15 min.
Add to each tube 0.5 ml of the 5 per cent rabbit erythrocytes suspension and shake well.

O-ANTISTREPTOLYSINS TITRATION PROTOCOL FOR DISTRIBUTION OF COMPONENTS

Tubes n°		1	2	3	4	5	6	7	8	9	10	11	12	(a)	(b)
Serum dilutions		1/10			1/100				1/500						
Serum	ml	0.8	0.2	1.0	0.8	0.6	0.4	0.3	1.0	0.8	0.6	0.4	0.2		
b s	ml	0.2	0.8	0.0	0.2	0.4	0.6	0.7	0.0	0.2	0.4	0.6	0.8	1.5	1.0
O-streptolysin (1 combining unit)	ml	0.5	0.5	0.5	0.5	0.5	0.5	0.5	0.5	0.5	0.5	0.5	0.5		0.5
O-antistreptolysins units		12	50	100	125	166	250	333	500	625	833	1250	2500		

Incubate at 37° C for 45 min, in water bath.

Centrifuge at 2,000 rpm for 1 min.

Read for results.

Interpretation of the results

The titer is given in antistreptolysin units by the tube in which total inhibition of hemolysis is produced by the highest dilution of serum.

Low titers (150 to 200 units) can be observed in normal sera.

Note: Commercial O-streptolysin, once dissolved in diluent, maintains its activity for at least 2 hr at room temperature (25° C).

19. TREPONEMA PALLIDUM [22] (Syphilis)

A number of tests are used in the diagnosis of syphilis. We shall describe shortly some of the most commonly used, referring to more complete sources for technical details.

Complement-fixation Test (Wassermann Test)

Antigens

(a) Treponemic antigen: Commercially available, it is prepared with Reiter's strain. It contains three antigenic components:

(1) treponemic, aspecific, ubiquitary, lipoid in nature;

(2) treponemic, specific, thermolabile, and

(3) treponemic, aspecific, thermoresistant.

(b) Cardiolipin: Commercially available, it is a phospholipid isolated from heart alcoholic extracts. It is alcohol soluble and acetone insoluble; contains 4 per cent phosphorus, no nitrogen. It is not fully reactive as such, as it needs the presence of purified lecithin and cholesterol.

Complement

Lyophilized complement is available commercially. It can be prepared by defibrinating the blood from young male fastened guinea pigs, after centrifugation at 3,000 rpm for 15 min. After two or three days storage at −20° C, the complement is titrated.

Sheep erythrocytes

Defibrinated sheep blood is washed three times in saline and then centrifuged at 3,000 rpm for 10 min. The sedimented erythrocytes are suspended in saline or in Alsever's solution to 5 per cent concentration.

Anti-sheep erythrocytes hemolysin

Commercially available.

Complement titration

To titrate the complement at a $\frac{1}{30}$ dilution, using 2 hemolytic units (HU), the following scheme is used:

Complement 1/30	ml	0.30	0.25	0.20	0.15	0.12	0.10
Saline	ml	0.20	0.25	0.30	0.35	0.38	0.40

Incubate in water bath at 37°C, for 1 hr.
Add:

Hemolysin 2 HU	ml	0.10	0.10	0.10	0.10	0.10	0.10
Sheep erythrocytes 2%	ml	0.10	0.10	0.10	0.10	0.10	0.10

Incubate in water bath at 37°C, for 1 hr.

Interpretation of the results

The smallest amount of complement able to produce a complete hemolysis represents 1 unit of complement.

The following scheme can be followed to dilute complement in order to obtain 2 units of complement in 0.20 ml:

1 Unit/ml	0.30	0.25	0.20	0.15	0.12	0.10
Dilution of the complement to obtain 2 U/0.20 ml:	1/10	1/12	1/15	1/20	1/25	1/30

Preparation of the hemolytic system

Mix 0.10 ml of commercial hemolysin with 9.9 ml of saline.
Mix 0.10 ml of the $\frac{1}{100}$ dilution of hemolysin with 9.0 ml of saline; store at 4° C the remaining $\frac{1}{100}$ dilution.
Dilute the $\frac{1}{1,000}$ hemolysin over, according to the following scheme:

Hemolysin 1/1,000 ml		1	1	1	1	1	1
Saline	ml	1	1.5	2.0	2.5	3.0	3.5
Final dilutions		1/2,000	1/2,500	1/3,000	1/3,500	1/4,000	1/4,500

And over, if necessary

To titrate the hemolysin, according to the Wassermann technique, use the following scheme:

Saline	ml	0.50	0.50	0.50	0.50	0.50	0.50	0.50
Sheep erythrocytes 5%	ml	0.25	0.25	0.25	0.25	0.25	0.25	0.25
Complement 1/10	ml	0.25	0.25	0.25	0.25	0.25	0.25	0.25
Hemolysin dilutions	ml	0.25	0.25	0.25	0.25	0.25	0.25	0.25
		1/1,000	1/2,000	1/2,500	1/3,000	1/3,500	1/4,000	1/4,500

Incubate at 37° C for 45 min.

To titrate the hemolysin, according to the Kolmer technique, use the following scheme:

Saline	ml	0.40	0.40	0.40	0.40	0.40	0.40	0.40
Sheep erythrocytes 2%	ml	0.10	0.10	0.10	0.10	0.10	0.10	0.10
Complement 1/30	ml	0.10	0.10	0.10	0.10	0.10	0.10	0.10
Hemolysin dilutions	ml	0.10	0.10	0.10	0.10	0.10	0.10	0.10
		1/1,000	1/2,000	1/2,500	1/3,000	1/3,500	1/4,000	1/4,500

Incubate at 37° C in water bath for 1 hr.
Read for results.

Interpretation of the results for hemolysin titration

The higher dilution of hemolysin, where complete hemolysis is obtained, represents the Hemolytic Unit (HU).

Hemolytic system

Mix equal volumes of sheep erythrocytes 5 per cent suspension and hemolysin dilutions containing respectively 2 HU for cardiolipin antigen, and 4 HU for treponemic antigen.
Incubate at 37° C for about 15 min.

Note: To obtain the desired number of hemolytic units, the hemolysin dilution should be respectively two and four times more concentrated than the one containing 1 HU.

Kolmer's technique

This technique differs from the other ones due to the fact that 2 units of complement are used with 2 units of hemolysin, for the use of a 2 per cent suspension of erythrocytes, and because the complement-fixation incubation time is 18 hr at 6 to 10° C.

Technique of the Wassermann test on serum

Inactivate the serum to be tested at 56° C for 30 min. A known negative serum is also tested as a control.

Dilute serum in saline (0.9 per cent) ⅕.

Place into three separate tubes, respectively 0.25 ml into the first two and 0.50 ml into the third, the diluted serum.

Add to the first tube 0.25 ml of the cardiolipin antigen and to the second one 0.25 ml of the treponemic antigen, both diluted according to the enclosed indications. The third tube is kept as a control for possible anticomplementary activity of the serum.

Add to all tubes 0.25 ml of complement dilution containing 2 units.

Prepare a control for each antigen, placing into two separate tubes 0.25 ml of saline, 0.25 ml of antigen, 0.25 ml of complement.

Shake well and incubate in water bath at 37° C for 45 min.

Note: At this point the hemolytic system is prepared as described above.

Add to all tubes 0.50 ml of the hemolysin-sheep erythrocytes mixture containing 2 HU.

Shake well and incubate in water bath at 37 °C until complete hemolysis is observed in all control tubes. At this point, it can be useful to put the tubes in cold water baths to stop the reaction.

Read for results.

Interpretation of the results

A complete hemolysis in all tubes is observed when the test

is negative. The lack of hemolysis in control tubes reveals the anticomplementary activity of some components of the reaction (serum, antigen, etc.).

Sometimes a slight anticomplementarity can be overcome by prolonging the incubation time.

The degree of positivity is indicated as follows:

+++ : no hemolysis
++ : 50 per cent hemolysis
+ : 75 per cent hemolysis
− : 100 per cent hemolysis

In the interpretation of the Wassermann test the following elements are kept into account for the diagnosis:

	Active Infection	Syphiloma or Old Infection or Recent Under Treatment	Congenital Infection or Aspecific Reaction	Negative
Cardiolipin antigen	+++	−	+++	−
Treponemic antigen	+++	+++	−	−

Technique of the Wassermann test on spinal fluid (sf)

Distribute in two sets of tubes 0.10, 0.20, 0.30, 0.40, 0.50 ml of undiluted sf (some authors suggest heating sf at 56° C for 15 min).

Add saline to all tubes to reach a volume of 0.50 ml.

Add to the first set of tubes 0.50 ml of the cardiolipin antigen and, to the second one, 0.50 ml of the treponemic antigen.

Prepare the same controls as described for the technique on serum.

Add to all tubes 0.50 ml of complement.

Incubate at 37° C in water bath for 1 hr.

Add to all tubes 1.0 ml of the hemolytic system, prepared as described above.

Incubate at 37° C in water bath for about 1 hr, or until hemolysis has taken place in the control tubes.

Read for results.

Interpretation of the results

The reaction is considered positive also when a complete inhibition of hemolysis is observed with just one of the two antigens and in the tube where the sf is more concentrated. In such cases, when only an incomplete hemolysis is observed, the result is negative. If a history of syphilitic infection is present, the result is dubious.

Venereal Diseases Research Laboratory (VDRL) Flocculation Test On Serum

Place into a container 0.40 ml of the diluent (commercially available).

Add drop by drop, with a new pipette, 0.50 ml of the antigen (commercially available), shaking the container thoroughly.

Add quickly 4.5 ml of the diluent, shaking the container thoroughly.

Place uniformly 0.05 ml of serum (heated at 56° C for 30 min), using a 0.1 ml pipette, at the bottom of a well.

Place one drop of the antigen on the serum by means of a syringe with a needle.

Rotate the slide at 120 rotations per min for 4 min, using a mechanical rotator.

To avoid evaporation, it is useful to place the slide into a Petri dish containing a piece of wet filter paper.

Read macroscopically against a dark surface and microscopically for results.

Interpretation of the results

+++: flocculation visible macroscopically
++: low flocculation visible macroscopically
+: uniform flocculation visible microscopically
+−: irregular flocculation visible microscopically
−: no flocculation

VDRL Flocculation Test On Spinal Fluid

Use the same technique described above (the sf should be absolutely clear and free from any trace of serum).

Wait 5 min after rotation before reading for results.

Kahn Test On Serum

Place into one tube 1.0 ml of the antigen (commercially available).

Place into a second tube an amount of saline according to the indications included.

Mix by pouring the saline into the tube containing the antigen and vice versa for six times.

Leave the mixture for 10 min and use it within 30 min.

Distribute the diluted antigen, using a 0.1 ml pipette, into three separate tubes, placing 0.05 ml into the first, 0.025 ml into the second and 0.0125 ml into the third.

Add to each tube 0.15 ml of the serum to be tested (heated at 56° C for 30 min).

Prepare two controls in the same way, using a known positive and a known negative serum.

Shake thoroughly for a few seconds.

Shake again for 3 min; a mechanical shaker can be used at 275 oscillations (4 cm range) per min.

Add 1.0 ml of saline into the first tube and 0.50 ml into the second and third.

Shake for a few seconds.

After 15 to 30 min,

Read for results.

A good reading is obtained holding the tubes inclined at 2 to 3 cm from the concavity of a microscope mirror placed on a table.

Interpretation of the results

++++: coarse granulations suspended in a clear fluid.

+++: finer granulations suspended in a rather turbid fluid.

++: fine granulations visible only with the help of a mirror or agglutinoscope.

+: very fine dusty-looking granulations visible with the help of a mirror or agglutinoscope.

+—: granulations visible just with the help of a mirror or agglutinoscope.

—: no granulations visible.

An average of the results observed in the three tubes is then made.

Tube n°	1	2	3	Average of Results
	++++	++++	++++	++++
	++	+++	++++	+++
	+	+++	++++	+++
	−	+++	++++	++
	−	++	++++	++
	−	+−	++++	+
	−	−	+++	+
	−	+−	+	−

Kahn Test On Spinal Fluid

Mix into a centrifuge tube 1.5 ml of clear sf with 1.5 ml of $(NH_4)_2SO_4$ saturated solution.

Shake the mixture thoroughly and heat it at 56° C for 15 min.

Centrifuge at 3,000 rpm for 5 to 10 min.

Prepare two controls, with known negative and known positive sf, in the same way.

Discard the supernatant; filter paper can be used for better results.

Resuspend the sediment in 0.15 ml of saline.

Place 0.15 ml of such suspension into a tube and add to it 0.01 ml of antigen prepared as described for the test on serum.

Shake thoroughly for 3 min with no interruptions.

Add 0.50 ml of saline.

Shake for 1 min.

After about 30 min,

Read for results.

Interpretation of the results

The results of the test are recorded as described for the test on serum.

Fluorescent antibody

The principle of the fluorescent antibody technique is based on the conjugation of an antibody protein with a fluorescent substance; the antigen-antibody reaction is then visualized by means of an ultraviolet source of light.

A direct test can be performed using a conjugated antiserum for each antigen to be tested. When dealing with a large number of antigens, the indirect method is more convenient; the antigen and the antibody are challenged and after repeated washings a conjugated gammaglobulin antiserum is stratified on the system.

If specific antibodies are present in the serum, they fix on the antigen despite washings and the anti-gammaglobulins antibodies fix on them and are demonstrable on ultraviolet observation. On the opposite, if no specific antibodies are present in the serum the anti-gammaglobulins will not fix themselves on the system and no fluorescence is obtained.

In some instances, a conjugated anti-guinea pig complement serum has been used on systems in which antigen, antibody, and complement were involved in the reaction.

Many fluorochromes have been used and experimented; the one more commonly employed is the fluorescein isothiocynate, due to the good stability and the low toxicity.

The fluorescent antibody technique has been used in all fields of immunology with great success for the relative simplicity and the practical results in research work.

Fluorescent Antibody Test in Syphilis

Antigen: lyophilized, commercially available. It is prepared from the Nichols strain of pathogenic treponemata.

Human antiglobulin: lyophilized, commercially available, conjugated with fluorescein isothiocynate.

Technique of the test

Dilute the lyophilized antigen with distilled H_2O, according to the indications.

Place 0.01 ml of the suspension on two separate points of a slide, marking the areas.

Dry the suspension at 37° C, placing the slide on a mechanical rotator at 100 rotations per min.

Immerse the slide in pure acetone in a Coplin dish for 10 min.

Let dry at room temperature.

Heat the serum to be tested in water bath at 56° C for 30 min.

Dilute serum in buffered solution (bs) (pH 7.2) $\frac{1}{50}$ and $\frac{1}{200}$
(serum 0.1 ml + bs 4.9 ml = $\frac{1}{50}$ → 1.0 ml + bs 3.0 ml = $\frac{1}{200}$).

Place 0.03 ml of the $\frac{1}{50}$ dilution of the serum on one of the two areas on which the treponemata suspension has been fixed and, using a new pipette, 0.03 ml of the $\frac{1}{200}$ dilution on the second area.

Place the slide into a Petri dish containing a piece of wet filter paper to avoid evaporation.

Incubate the Petri dish at 37° C for 30 min.

Remove the slide from the Petri dish and wash carefully in bs (pH 7.2).

Immerse the slide in bs for 10 min, renewing the fluid after 5 min.

Dry the slide carefully by means of filter paper.

Dilute the anti-human globulin in bs (pH 7.2) containing 2 per cent Tween-80, according to the indications enclosed.

Place 0.03 ml of the diluted antihuman gamma globulins on each area.

Place again in a Petri dish, prepared as described above, and incubate at 37° C for 30 min.

Wash and immerse in bs as described above.

Dry the slide carefully on filter paper.

Place a small drop of a 10 per cent bs in glycerin on the areas and cover with cover-glasses.

Repeat the procedure using a known negative and a known positive serum as controls.

Read for results, using a dark-field apparatus, first under normal and then under ultraviolet light.

Interpretation of the results

When the test is *negative,* the spirochetes, visible at dark-field examination under normal light, disappear or are hardly visible under ultraviolet light.

When the test is *positive,* the spirochetes are clearly visible under ultraviolet light, showing a greenish-yellow color.

It is important to notice that sometimes, due to a bad fixation on the slide, the concentration of organisms is poor; in such cases, it is advisable to repeat the whole procedure.

Note: It is worth mentioning the immobilization test on living spirochetes, developed by Nelson and Mayer, for its specificity and long duration in revealing the presence of antibodies.

20. VIBRIO CHOLERAE (Cholera)

Agglutinins appear about seven days after the onset of the disease and are detectable for about four to six months after recovery. This test has particular importance in epidemiological research.

Bacteriolysins appear later than agglutinins.

Preparation of the antigen and technique of the agglutination test

The antigen is prepared by suspending a loopful of a fresh growth of organism (Inaba, Ogawa strains) on agar, in ps.

One drop of the serum to be tested and one drop of the vibrios suspension are mixed on a slide.

Tilting the slide for 1 min, a uniform clumping of the vibrios is observed with positive sera.

21. COMPLEMENT-FIXATION TEST WITH BACTERIAL ANTIGENS [4]

The technique of the C-F test with bacterial antigens is similar to the standard one described on page 29. There is some difference in the titration of antigens. The serum, after inactivation at 56° C for 30 min, is incubated again at 37° C for 1 hr after addition of a small amount of concentrated sheep erythrocytes suspension to remove any residual anticomplementarity.

After incubation serum is centrifuged, an "anticomplementary" titration is performed to determine the anticomplementary unit, or the smallest amount of antigen having some inhibitory power on hemolysis.

Technique of the test

Prepare a set of ten serology tubes.

Add to each tube 0.50 ml of undiluted antigen and diluted $\frac{1}{2}$, $\frac{1}{3}$, $\frac{1}{4}$, $\frac{1}{6}$, $\frac{1}{8}$, $\frac{1}{10}$, $\frac{1}{12}$, $\frac{1}{16}$, $\frac{1}{20}$, respectively.

Add to each tube 0.50 ml of ps and 2 units of complement in
1.0 ml.

Prepare the following controls:

(a) place into one tube 1.0 ml of saline for hemolytic control, and

(b) place into a second tube 2.5 ml of saline for erythrocytes
control.

Refrigerate at 4° C for 2 hr or overnight.

Incubate in water bath at 37° C for 30 min.

Add to all tubes, but (b), 0.5 ml of hemolysin, containing 2 HU.

Add to all tubes, and to control tubes (a) and (b), 0.50 ml of a
2 per cent suspension of erythrocytes in saline.

Incubate in water bath at 37° C for 1 hr.

Interpretation of the results

The anticomplementary unit is given by the smallest amount
of antigen having some inhibitory power on hemolysis. Control
(a) should show complete hemolysis; control (b), no hemolysis.

Following the anticomplementary titration, an antigenic titration is performed.

Prepare a set of nine serology tubes.

Add to each tube 0.50 ml of the following dilutions of the an-
tigen: $\frac{1}{10}$, $\frac{1}{20}$, $\frac{1}{40}$, $\frac{1}{60}$, $\frac{1}{80}$, $\frac{1}{100}$, $\frac{1}{200}$, $\frac{1}{300}$, $\frac{1}{400}$.

Add to each tube 0.50 ml of known, undiluted, positive serum.

Add to each tube 2 units of complement in 1.0 ml.

Prepare the following controls:

(a) ps 0.50 ml; complement 1.0 ml; positive serum 0.50 ml;

(b) ps 1.0 ml; complement 1.0 ml;

(c) ps 2.5 ml.

Incubate at 4° C for 2 hr or overnight.

Incubate at 37° C for 30 min.

Add to all tubes, and to control tubes (a) and (b), hemolysin
and erythrocytes suspension as in the anticomplementary titration test.

Add to control tube (c) only 0.50 ml of the erythrocytes suspension.

Incubate at 37° C for 1 hr.

Interpretation of the results

The antigenic unit is the smallest amount of antigen giving a 4+ result. In control tubes (a) and (b), a complete hemolysis should be observed, in control tube (c), no hemolysis.

An antigen may be used in the amount equivalent to about one-third or one-fourth of its anticomplementary unit. To obtain it practically, multiply the dilutions by three or four.

BIBLIOGRAPHY

1. CASTAÑEDA, M. R.: In, GRADWOHL, *Clinical Laboratory Methods and Diagnosis*. Frankel and Reitman Ed., Sixth Ed., St. Louis, C. V. Mosby Co., 1963, Vol. 1, p. 760.
2. CASTAÑEDA, M. R., SILVA, R., and MONNIER, A.: *Rev Med Hosp Gen*, 2:382, 1940.
3. CRAVITZ, I., and MILLER, W. R.: *J Infect Dis*, 86:46, 1950.
4. GRADWOHL: *Clinical Laboratory Methods and Diagnosis*. Frankel and Reitman Ed., Sixth Ed., St. Louis, C. V. Mosby Co., 1963, Vol. 1, p. 772.
5. GRADWOHL (revised by FELSENFELD, O.): *Clinical Laboratory Methods and Diagnosis*, E. Kimpton, Fifth Ed., London, 1956, Vol. 2, p. 1,562.
6. GREENWALD, E.: *JAMA, 121*:9, 1943.
7. HODGE, B. E., and SWIFT, H. F.: *J Exp Med, 58*:277, 1933.
8. KALBAK, K.: *Ejnar Munksgaards Forlag*. Kobenhavn, 1942.
9. MACKIE, T. T., HUNTER, G. W., and WORTH, C. B.: *A Manual of Tropical Medicine*, Second Ed., Philadelphia and London, W. B. Saunders Co., 1955, p. 129.
10. MARTIN, L., and PETTIT, A.: *Serodiagnostico de la L.i.h.*, 2:1,121, 1918.
11. McFARLAND, J.: *JAMA, 49*:1,176, 1907.
12. NJOKU-OBI, A. N.: *Cornell Vet, 52*:415, 1962.
13. NUNGESTER, W. J.: In, DUBOS, R. J.: *Bacterial and Mycotic Infections of Man*. Second Ed., Philadelphia and Montreal, J. B. Lippincott Co., 1952, p. 378.
14. POWELL, H. M., and JAMIESON, W. A.: *J Immun, 43*:13, 1942.
15. QUINN, R. W., and LIAO, S. J.:*J Clin Invest, 29*:1,156, 1950.
16. RANTZ, L. A., DI CAPRIO, J. M., and RANDALL, E.: *Am J Med, 224*:194, 1952.

17. RANTZ, L. A., and RANDALL, E.: *Proc Soc Exp Biol Med* (N.Y.), 59:22, 1945.

18. RANTZ, L. A., RANDALL, E., and RANTZ, H. H.: *Amer J Med,* 5:3, 1948.

19. SCHAUB, I. G., and FOLEY, M. K.: *Diagnostic Bacteriology.* London, H. Kimpton, 1952, p. 267.

20. *Ibid.,* p. 270.

21. SCHUEFFNER, W., and BOLHANDER, H.: *Zbl Bakt, I. Abt Orig, 144:* 434, 1939.

22. SCLAVO, S. P. A.: Istituto Sieroterapico e Vaccinogeno Toscano, Siena (Italia), Technical notes.

23. SONNENWIRTH, A. C.: In, GRADWOHL, *Clinical Laboratory Methods and Diagnosis.* Frankel and Reitman Ed., Sixth Ed., St. Louis, C. V. Mosby Co., 1963, Vol. 1, p. 760.

24. TODD, E. W.: *J Exp Med,* 55:267, 1932.

25. ZANGAGLIA, O., and CAMBIERI, F.: In, INTROZZI, P., *Trattato Italiano di Medicina Interna, Tecniche e Diagnostica di Laboratorio.* Roma, Abruzzini Ed., 1960, Vol. 3, p. 2,084.

26. *Ibid.,* p. 2,085.

27. *Ibid.,* p. 2,102.

28. *Ibid.,* p. 2,111.

29. *Ibid.,* p. 2,114.

30. *Ibid.,* p. 2,140.

31. *Ibid.,* p. 2,157.

32. ZARDI, O.: *Nuovi Ann Ig Microbiol,* 14:165, 1963.

II

SEROLOGICAL DIAGNOSTIX IN PARASITIC DISEASES

1. ECHINOCOCCUS GRANULOSUS [12, 13, 14]
(Hydatid Disease)

T<small>HE</small> E<small>CHINOCOCCOSIS</small> complement-fixation test is performed following the same technique described for syphilis. (See page 29.)

The antigen used is the cystic fluid drawn and preserved under sterile conditions.

Complement-fixation (C-F) Test [2] (Ghedini-Weinberg Test)

PROTOCOL FOR COMPLEMENT-FIXATION TEST IN ECHINOCOCCOSIS

Tubes n°		1	2	3	4 Contr.	5 Contr.
Serum 56°C/30°	ml	0.10	0.10	0.10	0.10	
Cystic fluid	ml	0.50	0.25	0.10		0.50
Ps	ml	0.40	0.65	0.80	0.90	0.50
Complement (1/10)	ml	0.50	0.50	0.50	0.50	0.50
		Incubate at 37°C in water bath for 1 hr.				
Hemolytic system	ml	1.0	1.0	1.0	1.0	1.0
		Incubate at 37°C in water bath until hemolysis in control tubes				

Interpretation of the results

Hemolysis is read as in the Wassermann test. Inhibition of hemolysis in the three tubes containing serum dilutions is considered strong positivity; if inhibition of hemolysis is observed in two tubes, the response is positive; if in only one tube, the first, lack of hemolysis is obtained, the result is recorded as weak positivity.

Sometimes the test may be negative in cases of echinococcosis; aspecific responses are rather rare.

The presence of cysts, after surgery, can be revealed by persistent positivity of C-F tests.

Precipitation Test[2] (Fleige and Lisbonne Test)

Place into a serology tube 0.5 ml of serum to be tested.
Add 0.5 ml of cyst fluid.
Shake well at 37° C for 2 hr.
Read for results.

Interpretation of the results

In about 20 per cent of echinococcosis cases, a precipitate can be observed.

2. LEISHMANIA DONOVANI[5] (Visceral Leishmaniasis, Kala-Azar)

Complement-fixation Test

This test is not commonly used for the presence of group-reactions.

Antigen is prepared from leishmanias washed and centrifuged in saline. After the washing procedure, acetone is added to the bulk of organisms and stored for a few days at 4° C. When the acetone evaporates, the antigen is triturated and extracted in ethyl alcohol.

Also, a tubercle antigen, nonspecific, has proved useful in the C-F test.

Note: Nonantibody-antigen reaction tests are used in L. donovani infections:

Formol-gel Test[6]

Add one drop of 40 per cent commercial formaldehyde to 1.0 ml of the serum to be tested, into a serology tube.

Interpretation of the results

In positive sera, coagulation occurs within 1 hr. In patients affected by Kala-Azar, the reaction takes place in a few seconds. In American visceral leishmaniasis, the reaction is slow during the first period of the disease and the velocity increases as it progresses.

In other diseases, such as malaria, leprosy, alastrim, etc., the reaction takes a long time.

Brahmachari Test[6]

Place 1.0 ml of the serum to be tested in a serology tube.
Flow 2 to 3.0 ml of distilled H_2O along the walls of the tube.

Interpretation of the results

In positive sera, due to the increase of globulin and the reduction of albumin, a turbid ring forms at the point of contact of distilled H_2O and serum.

This test is not specific and may be observed in malaria as well.

3. TOXOPLASMA GONDII[23] (Toxoplasmosis)

Neutralization Test on Rabbit[20] (Sabin and Ruchman Test)

This test is not very widely used at the present.

Serum: Freshly drawn (not over 24 hr) or after storage at $-20°$ C to preserve the "accessory activator factor." If the serum is more than 24 hr old or has not been stored at $-20°$ C, it can be used after addition of fresh human serum, free of specific antibodies.

Rabbit: White rabbit, shaved on his sides. One rabbit is sufficient to test four sera.

Mark one row of five points for every serum to be tested and one row for controls.

Toxoplasma suspension: A toxoplasma suspension is obtained by grounding and suspending $1/10$ in sterile saline, an animal brain rich of agents and kept at $4°$ C for 1 hr to sediment. The suspension is then diluted in sterile saline to obtain $1/10$, $1/50$, $1/500$, $1/1,500$ concentrations.

Intraperitoneal exudate, rich in toxoplasma, can be used at the same dilutions.

Technique of the test

Add to 0.20 ml of the toxoplasma suspension an equal amount of serum to be tested, and an equal amount of saline for the controls. The final dilution of the suspension is now $\frac{1}{20}$, $\frac{1}{100}$, $\frac{1}{1,000}$, $\frac{1}{10,000}$.

Inoculate subcutaneously, on the marked points 0.20 ml of the serum-suspension mixtures, starting cranially with the highest dilution and using the same syringe, except for the control row.

Interpretation of the results

After about one week, erythematous lesions showing a central necrosis will be observed in the points of inoculation. The lesions will be more severe where the more concentrated suspensions have been inoculated. If the serum contains specific antibodies, the difference among the serum-suspension and the control lesions will be evident.

Dye Test [19] (Sabin and Feldman Test)

The action of specific neutralizing antibodies on toxoplasma produces some changes in the cytoplasm behavior towards vital dyes.

Toxoplasma, under normal conditions, is well stained with methylene blue solutions and the oval or slightly curved shape is well maintained.

On the contrary, after incubation with specific neutralizing antibodies, the affinity for dyes is lost and, as the nucleus is stained, the cytoplasm is not. Morphologically, the organisms appear thinner and sickle-shaped.

Serum: The serum, if freshly drawn, should be inactivated at 56° C for 30 min in order to destroy the "activator factor." When dilution is performed or when serum has been stored for a period of time, such factor is destroyed and heating is no longer necessary. It is preferable, in any case, to heat all sera to avoid possible discrepancies in the results.

Technique of the test

Prepare two-fold dilutions of the serum to be tested and of positive and negative control sera in saline, beginning from $\frac{1}{2}$ up to $\frac{1}{1,024}$, or over, if necessary (for routine work $\frac{1}{16}$, $\frac{1}{64}$, $\frac{1}{256}$ dilutions are sufficient).

Mix 1 volume of peritoneal exudate (mice are used)* with $\frac{1}{10}$ volume of heparin 1 per cent solution. Add to this mixture 4 volumes of human normal fresh or lyophilized serum, free of antibodies (i.e., peritoneal exudate 0.20 ml, heparin 0.02 ml, serum 0.80 ml).

Add 0.10 ml of the mixture to all tubes containing sera dilutions. Incubate in water bath at 37° C for 1 hr.

Mix on a slide one drop of each serum dilution with one drop of methylene blue solution.†

Place cover glasses on slides and read for staining at high dry magnification under a microscope.

Interpretation of the results

One hundred organisms are counted for staining results. The serum dilution, in which 50 per cent of unstained toxoplasma are observed, represents the antibody titer of the serum.

Complement-fixation Test[16] (Nicolau and Ravelo-Sabin)

Preparation of the antigen

Prepare a 10 per cent suspension of toxoplasma infected mouse brain in sterile physiological saline.

Inoculate 0.10 ml of such suspension in ten-day-old embryonated eggs.

Incubate for six more days: triturate chorioallantoic membranes in a mortar with quartz sand.

Suspend in ps buffered to pH 7.5 to 10 per cent concentration.

Freeze and thaw three times consecutively and centrifuge at 13,000 rpm.

Transfer the supernatant to a new container, add Merthiolate to a $\frac{1}{10,000}$ concentration.

Store at −20° C until used.

---

* To prepare the toxoplasma suspension, inoculate mice intraperitoneally with a virulent strain of toxoplasma. Draw the exudate after 2 to 3 days.

† Prepare extemporally the methylene blue solution by mixing

Na_2CO_3	0.53 per cent in distilled H_2O	9.73 ml
$Na_2B_4O_7$	1.91 per cent in distilled H_2O	0.27 ml
Methylene blue alcoholic (95 per cent) saturated solution (pH 11.0).		3.0 ml

Technique of the test

See technique on page 29. (Two Hemolytic Units [HU] are employed.)

Hemagglutination Test[10]

Preparation of the antigen

Dilute mouse peritoneal exudate in buffered physiological saline (bps), (pH 7.0), and centrifuge in graduated tube at 1,500 rpm for 5 min.

Discard the supernatant and add distilled H_2O ten times the humid sediment weight.

Shake well and store at 4° C for 20 hr with frequent shaking.

Centrifuge again.

Mix equal volumes of the supernatant and NaCl 1.7 per cent solution.

Distribute in several small, sterile containers and store at −20° C until used.

Preparation of the sheep erythrocytes

Mix 0.50 ml of washed sheep erythrocytes with 20.0 ml of tannic acid $\frac{1}{20,000}$ solution and 19.5 ml of bps (pH 7.2).

Incubate in water bath at 37° C for 10 min.

Centrifuge at 1,000 rpm for 5 min.

Discard the supernatant and resuspend sediment in 30.0 ml of bps (pH 7.2).

Centrifuge again, discard, and resuspend in 20.0 ml.

Mix the erythrocytes suspension with 20.0 ml of $\frac{1}{50}$ diluted antigen and 60.0 ml of bps (pH 6.4).

Keep at room temperature for 15 min.

Centrifuge at 1,000 rpm for 5 min.

Discard the supernatant and wash three or four times the sediment in $\frac{1}{250}$ diluted human normal serum.

Resuspend the erythrocytes sediment in 19.5 ml of normal human serum ($\frac{1}{250}$).

Technique of the test

Prepare two-fold dilutions of sera in normal human serum ($\frac{1}{100}$), beginning from ½ up to $\frac{1}{512}$, or over.

Distribute 0.50 ml of each dilution into serology tubes.

Replace, for control, serum dilution with saline.

Add, to each tube, 0.10 ml of sensitized erythrocytes suspension.

Incubate at 4° C for 18 hr.

Read for results.

Interpretation of the results

The antibody titer of the serum is given by the highest dilution in which hemagglutination is observed.

4. TRICHINELLA SPIRALIS (Trichinosis)

Several tests have been developed for the serologic diagnosis of trichinosis. The preparation of antigens is rather complicated, and in some instances we shall refer directly to the original works.[9]

Preparation of the antigens [1]

1) Crude antigen extract:

Feed rats of an average weight of 150.0 gm four thousand viable larvae of T. spiralis.

After four weeks, sacrifice the animals and grind the skinned and eviscerated carcasses.

Take[7] a 3 liter capacity funnel, the stem of which is connected to a centrifuge tube by a rubber tube, and provide it with a 6 in perforated porcelain plate. Place four or five layers of cheesecloth over this plate. The cheesecloth should have about forty mesh apertures to the inch.

Prepare digestive fluid by dissolving 10.0 gm of pepsin/1 liter distilled H_2O, and add 7.0 ml of hydrochloric acid (sp g 1.10 to 1.19).

Pour digestive fluid into the funnel and gently add the ground carcasses.

Incubate at 37° C for 18 hr.

Clip the rubber tube and remove the centrifuge tube.

Remove the sediment containing larvae.

Wash the larvae four times in ps, changing the tube after each washing and having let the larvae sediment.

Perform a biuret test on the fourth supernatant and, if positive,
   wash again; if negative,
Add 2.0 ml of larvae bulk to 8.0 ml of saline and grind in a Ten
   Broeck grinder.
Bring to 40.0 ml with saline.
Keep at room temperature for 3 hr.
Keep at 4° C for 12 hr.
Centrifuge at 10,000 g for 30 min and discard the sediment.
Centrifuge again.
Add Merthiolate to a $\frac{1}{10,000}$ dilution.
Store at 4° C. If stored at −20° C, will maintain up to three years.

   Note: In centrifuge operations either "revolutions per minute"
(rpm) or "relative centrifugal forces" (RCF) or gravities (g)
are indicated.

   Rpm are given on centrifuges by ordinary indicators; to calculate RCF the following equation is used:

RCF: $0.00001118 \times r \times N^2$

RCF = relative centrifugal forces (gravities).
   r = rotating radius (in centimeters).
   N = rotating speed (in rpm).

The following equations can also be used:

RCF: $0.0000284 \times r \times N^2$ (when calculated in inches).
RCF: $(11.1787) \ 10^{-6} \times r \times N^2$ (when calculated in centi-
meters).
For quick computation of values nomographs can be used.

2) Melcher's antigen: [15]

   This method of preparing Trichinella antigen is very simple.

   Through a Soxhlet apparatus, 2 gm of lyophilized powdered
larvae are extracted for seven days with petroleum ether.
   The temperature is adjusted to allow the apparatus to empty
every 15 min.
   The larvae, once removed from the ether, are extracted for
about 12 hr at 4° C in borate buffer (pH 8.3). The extract is then
centrifuged at 10,000 g for 30 min and the supernatant is stored

at 4° C, after the pH has been brought to 4.8 with 0.2N HCl. After centrifugation, remove precipitate; the clear supernatant is stored at −20° C before used as antigen.

Bentonite Flocculation Test[11]

Preparation of stock bentonite particles

In a Waring blendor, homogenize 0.5 gm of N°200 Standard Vol-
    clay ‡ in 100.0 ml of glass-distilled H_2O.
Bring the suspension to 500.0 ml with glass-distilled H_2O.
Shake and leave the suspension to rest for 1 hr.
Centrifuge the supernatant at 500 g for 15 min.
Decant the supernatant.
Centrifuge again at 700 g for 15 min.
Discard the supernatant.
Resuspend the sediment in 100.0 ml of glass-distilled H_2O, using
    a Waring blendor, for 1 min.
Store at 4° C.
    Note: If lyophilized Bentonite particles are used, some modi-
fications are employed in the technique.

Stock antigen

Shake the stock Bentonite suspension thoroughly.
Mix 20.0 ml of the suspension to 10.0 ml of T. spiralis antigen.
Mix well and store at 4° C for about 12 hr.
Add 5.0 ml of a 0.1 per cent thionin blue O water solution, and
    leave for 1 hr.
The stock antigen is stored at 4° C up to three months.

Test antigen

Shake the stock antigen thoroughly and transfer 8.0 ml of it to a
    centrifuge tube.
Wash twice by centrifugation at 1,000 g for 5 min, using 10 ml
    of saline.
Resuspend the sediment in 4.0 ml of saline.
Add 0.1 ml of Tween-80 solution (Tween-80, 0.5 ml, distilled
    H_2O, 99.5 ml) to the antigen and shake.

---

    ‡ Wyoming Bentonite.

Preliminary test of the antigen

Perform a flocculation test challenging the antigen with normal serum ($\frac{1}{100}$) and saline separately. If flocculation appears, more Tween-80 solution is added until a negative response is obtained with normal serum and less than the 50 per cent of the particles in saline are flocculated.

Perform two more flocculation tests using two positive control sera, one of high and one of low titer, to determine if there is an excess of Tween-80. If the positivity is more than one dilution lower than the given titer of the sera, antigen should be washed again in saline, centrifuged, resuspended and tested all over again, employing smaller amounts of Tween-80 solution.

Store the standardized antigen at 4° C up to one month.

Technique of the test

Inactivate serum to be tested at 56° C for 30 min.

Dilute serum in saline $\frac{1}{5}$, $\frac{1}{10}$, $\frac{1}{20}$, or over, if necessary.

Prepare the following controls:

(a) Positive inactivated serum and   for antigen activity
(b) Negative inactivated serum   and specificity
(c) Replace serum with saline for autoflocculation.

Place 0.1 ml of serum to be tested, the control sera and saline, on wax-ringed slides.

Add one drop of standardized test antigen, using a pipette delivering ±70 drops/ml.

Agitate slides on a rotating shaker at 100 rotations per min for 15 min.

Read microscopically for flocculation.

Note:

4+ = 100 per cent flocculated particles
3+ = 75 per cent flocculated particles
2+ = 50 per cent flocculated particles
1+ = 25 per cent flocculated particles

Complement-fixation Test

Several methods have been experimented for C-F testing in trichinosis. The Rees and Bozicevich method is suggested.[18]

Hemagglutination Test [12, 17, 21]

This test is still in an experimental stage and, though very promising, is not routinely used.

Latex Agglutination Test [8, 22]

Preparation of the stock suspension of Latex particles (0.81 μ diameter)

Dilute the original suspension with distilled H_2O until 0.1 ml of it, mixed with 10.0 ml of distilled H_2O, matches a light transmission of 5 per cent in a Coleman Un. spectrophotometer (model 11 or 14) in a square cuvet 13 x 13 x 100 mm at 650 mμ and a red filter.

Store at 4° C up to several months.

Technique of the test

Mix 4.0 ml of saline glycine buffer (pH 9.2) with 1.0 ml of T. spiralis antigen and 2.0 ml of Latex particles suspension.

Set a two-fold dilution of the serum to be tested.

Prepare the following controls:
  (a) Positive serum dilutions, and   for antigen activity
  (b) Negative serum dilutions   and specificity
  (c) Replace serum with glycine buffer for autoagglutination.
  (d) Replace the antigen with glycine buffer for autoagglutination.

Add 0.1 ml of antigen particles suspension (mind the antigen control) to all serology tubes containing 0.1 ml of serial dilutions of sera.

Incubate at 37° C for 30 min.

Cool at room temperature.

Centrifuge at 2,000 rpm for 3 min.

Read for results.

Interpretation of the results

Values of positivity are calculated as for flocculation. Positive tubes show flocculates and a clear supernatant; negative tubes show no flocculation and a cloudy supernatant.

5. TRYPANOSOMA CRUZI [4] (Chagas' Disease)

Complement-fixation Test

Preparation of the antigen (Kelser)

Cultivate T. cruzi in Kelser's medium.

Add 0.75 ml of sterile distilled H_2O to each culture tube.

Suspend the surface growth by means of a sterile glass pipette.

Transfer the suspension to a 15 ml graduated conical centrifuge tube.

Centrifuge at 4,000 g for 30 min.

Discard the supernatant.

Add 8.0 ml of sterile ps.

Centrifuge and wash twice again; eventually discard the supernatant.

Add 2 volumes of 50 per cent glycerin in ps.

Mix gently with a sterile glass rod.

Store at 4° C.

Technique of the test

The usual C-F technique is employed.

Note: Other types of antigens have been prepared as by extraction with ether and alkaline saline. To avoid cross-reaction with syphilitic and normal sera, a chloroform-gel technique has been developed, capable of separating specifically reactive proteins and carbohydrate antigens from aqueous extracts of ether-treated trypanosomes.

6. TRYPANOSOMA GAMBIENSE—RHODESIENSE

(African Trypanosomiasis)

In the diagnosis of trypanosomiasis, serological reactions are not widely used. The demonstration of agents in peripheral blood, or in other body fluids, remains the method of choice.

Adhesion Test[3]

A known, positive antiserum is used to titrate the guinea pig complement, the concentration of human erythrocytes, and the trypanosomes suspension to use in further tests.

The four components of the reaction—the serum to be tested, the trypanosomes suspension, the complement, and the human erythrocytes—are mixed at the optimal concentrations.

Interpretation of the results

The positive sera cause the adhesion of the erythrocytes and trypanosomes.

The test, however, is not generally used.

BIBLIOGRAPHY

1. BOZICEVICH, J.: *Public Health Rep, 53:*2,130, 1938.
2. FERRATA, A., and MEDURI, D.: In, INTROZZI, P.: *Trattato Italiano di Medicina Interna—Tecniche e Diagnostica di Laboratorio,* Abruzzini Ed., 1960, Vol. 3, p. 2,027.
3. GRADWOHL: *Clinical Laboratory Methods and Diagnosis.* Fifth Ed., London, H. Kimpton, 1956, Vol. 2, p. 1872.
4. *Ibid.,* p. 1,874.
5. GRADWOHL: *Clinical Laboratory Methods and Diagnosis.* Frankel and Reitman Ed., Sixth Ed., St. Louis, C. V. Mosby Co., 1963, Vol. 1, p. 903.
6. *Ibid.,* p. 1,022.
7. HOBMAIER, M., and MEYER, K. F.: *Science, 86:*568, 1937.
8. INELLA, F., and REDNER, W. J.: *JAMA, 171:*885, 1959.
9. KAGAN, I. G.: *J Infect Dis, 107:*69, 1960.
10. JACOBS, L., and LUNDE, M. N.: *Science, 125:*3,256, 1957.
11. KAGAN, I. G., ALLAIN, D. S., and NORMAN, L.: *Amer J Trop Med,* 8:51, 1959.
12. KAGAN, I. G., and BARGAI, V. J.: *Parasitology, 42:*237, 1956.
13. KAGAN, I. G., NORMAN, L., and ALLAIN, D. S.: *Amer J Trop Med,* 9:248, 1960.
14. MAGATH, T. B.: *J Clin Path, 31:*1, 1959.
15. MELCHER, L. R.: *J Infect Dis, 73:*31, 1943.

16. NICOLAU, S., and RAVELO, A.: *Bull Soc Path Exot, 30:*855, 1937.
17. PRICE, S. G., and WEINER, L. M.: *Amer J Clin Path, 26:*1,261, 1956.
18. REES, C. W., BOZICEVICH, J., REARDON, L. V., and JONES, F.: *Amer J Trop Med, 22:*581, 1942.
19. SABIN, A. B., and FELDMAN, H. A.: *Science, 85:*336, 1937.
20. SABIN, A. B., and RUCHMAN, J.: *Proc Soc Exp Biol Med, 51:*1, 1942.
21. SADUN, E. H., and ALLAIN, D. S.: *J Parasit, 43:*383, 1957.
22. SINGER, J. M., and PLOTZ, C. M.: *Amer J Med, 21:*888, 1956.
23. ZARDI, O.: *Nuovi Ann Ig Microbiol, 14:*491, 1963.

III

SEROLOGICAL DIAGNOSTIX IN MYCOTIC DISEASES

1. BLASTOMYCES DERMATITIDIS [2] (Blastomycosis)

Complement-fixation Test

Preparation of the antigen

Blastomycin can be used as antigen. It is prepared by the filtration of filamentous cultures grown in synthetic media. An antigen can also be prepared from the yeast phase of the organism.

Technique of the test

Usual C-F technique is used.

Interpretation of the results

Same as further for Histoplasmosis. Cross-reactions with Histoplasma are often observed, and also, to a lesser degree, with Coccidiomycosis and S. American blastomycosis.

Agglutination Test

An agglutination test, employing the standard technique, can be performed using blastomycin as an antigen.

2. HISTOPLASMA CAPSULATUM [1, 3, 4, 5] (Histoplasmosis)

Complement-fixation Test

Preparation of the antigen

Standard histoplasmin can be used as antigen. It is prepared by growing the organism at room temperature for two to four months and standardizing sterile filtrates.

An antigen can also be prepared from the yeast phase of the organism.

Technique of the test

Usual C-F technique is employed.

Interpretation of the results

Titers are low and must be interpreted on the basis of the entire clinical picture, and on the results of the histoplasmin skin test. Cross-reactions with Blastomyces and Coccidioides antigens are frequently observed. For this reason, the C-F test should always be performed with the three antigens at the same time for control.

BIBLIOGRAPHY

1. Furcolow, M. L.: *New Eng J Med, 286:*357, 1963.
2. Gradwohl: *Clinical Laboratory Methods and Diagnosis,* Frankel and Reitman Ed., Sixth Ed., St. Louis, C. V. Mosby Co., 1963, Vol. 1, p. 1,045.
3. *Ibid.,* p. 1,047.
4. Hill, G. B., and Campbell, C. C.: *J Lab Clin Med, 48:*255, 1956.
5. Saslaw, S., and Campbell, C. C.: *Proc Soc Exp Biol Med, 82:* 698, 1953.

IV

SEROLOGICAL DIAGNOSTIX IN VIRAL AND RICKETTSIAL DISEASES

1. PREPARATION OF VIRAL ANTIGENS

MANY METHODS are used in the preparation of viral antigens depending on the type of tissues in which viruses multiply.

Antigens can be prepared from viruses multiplying in cell cultures, in infected animal tissues or in fluids and tissues from infected embryonated eggs. They can be utilized living or inactivated, which is better for the safety of laboratory personnel.

Antigens can be purified and concentrated in many different ways.

In order to give good antigens, the original virus strains must reach high titers of activity, usually over 10^{-6}. While giving a list of the most common media for preparing antigens, as far as the particular techniques go, we make reference to the abundant literature easily found on the subject.

2. COMPLEMENT-FIXATION TEST [10, 16, 22]

Serum

Inactivate serum at 56° C for 30 min and, for long periods, store at −20° C, −30° C, and at 4° C if just for a few days. In order to avoid possible anticomplementarity of sera stored at −20° C, it is useful to thaw them about 20 hr before use, or to incubate again at 56°C for 10 to 15 min.

SEROLOGICAL METHODS FOR THE DIAGNOSIS OF THE MOST COMMON VIRUS DISEASES[1, 21, 29]

VIRUS	Preferable Source of Antigen for...	C-F Test	H A I Test	Test Species and...	Route of Inoculation for	Neutralization Test
Coxsackie						
A$_1$ to A$_{10}$	suckling mice torsos	+	7 +	suckling mice	subcutaneous (s c)	+
A$_{12-14-16-17-19-21\ to\ 24}$	idem	++	21,24 +	idem	s c	++
B$_1$ to B$_6$	idem, HeLa	++	20 +	idem, HeLa	s c	++
	FL, ammion, monkey kidneys (m k)	+	1,3,5 +	tissue cultures (t c)		+
ECHO						
1 to 20, 22 to 24, 26-27	m k	++++	3,6,7,11,12,13 19,20,24 +	t c		++++
21-25	HeLa, FL amnion	+++	21 +	t c		+++
Poliovirus 1-2-3	m k, human heart, etc.	++		t c		+
Adenovirus 1 to 28	K B HeLa	+	12-18 −	t c		++
C.C.A.	HeLa	+		HeLa		+
Influenza						
A – B	allantoic fluid	++	++	chick embryo, t c	allantoic	+++
C	idem	++	++	chick embryo	allantoic	++
Parainfluenza						
1 Sendai-H.A. 2	allantoic fluid, m k	+++	+++	chick embryo	allantoic	+++
2 C.A.	idem	+++	+++	idem	idem	+++
3 H.A. 1	idem			idem	idem	
Reovirus						
1 Lang, SV12	m k	++++	+++	m k		++++
2 D5, SV59	idem	+++	+++	idem		+++
3 Dearing, Abney	K B	++		K B		
R.S.V.	K B			K B		+
L.C.M.	mouse brain, guinea pig spleen and lungs	+		mouse, guinea pig	intracerebral (i c) s c	+
Mumps	allantoic fluid, chick embryo amnion cells, m k, HeLa	++	+++	chick embryo	amniotic	++
Variola	chorioallantoic membranes	++	+++	chick embryo	chorioallantoic	++
Vaccinia	MAF			MAF		++
Varicella	m k	+		m k		
Herpes zoster						

	chorioallantoic membranes		chick embryo	chorioallantoic	
Herpes simplex	+	+	chick embryo m k, human amnios cells		+ ± + +
Psittacosis Ornitosis Lymphogranuloma venereum	mouse spleen, yolk sac	+	chick embryo	yolk sac	+ +
Cat scratch fever	yolk sac	+	mouse	intranasal i c	+ +
Measles	K B, Hep 2, h. amnios cells	+	chick embryo, K B, Hep 2, h. amnios cells	yolk sac	+
(cross-reactions are observed with psittacosis-lymphogranuloma group antigens)					
Eastern equine encephalitis	mouse brain, amniotic, allantoic fluids and membranes	+	mouse	i c	+
St. Louis encephalitis	idem, chorioallantoic membranes	+	idem, HeLa	i c	+
Venezuelan equine encephalitis	mouse brain, amniotic, allantoic fluids and membranes	+	mouse	i c	+
Western equine encephalitis	idem	+	idem	i c	+
Japanese B encephalitis	mouse brain	+	idem	idem	+
Murray Valley encephalitis	idem	+	idem	idem	+
Central European encephalitis	idem, pig kidney cells (adapted strains)	+ +	idem	idem	+
Louping Ill	mouse brain, Detroit 6	+ +	idem, Detroit 6, HeLa	idem	+ +
Russian encephalitis	idem	+	idem	idem	+ +

Note: The table is not complete of all the serological methods available, as it schematizes the more common means used in the diagnosis of the principal virus diseases.

Hemolysin titration

(a) Distribute 0.40 ml of veronal buffer solution * (vbs) in eight rows of nine serology tubes each, in order to substitute antigen and antiserum.

Dilute hemolysin to $1/100$.

(b) Set up eight tubes and distribute, starting from the second one, 2.0 ml of vbs.

Distribute 2.0 ml of the hemolysin dilution in the first and second tubes.

Beginning from the second tube, after mixing well, pass 2.0 ml to the third tube, mix well again and pass 2.0 ml to the fourth, and so on to the eighth tube from which 2.0 ml are discarded. The hemolysin dilutions will now be equal to $1/100$, $1/200$, . . . $1/12,800$.

Add to the hemolysin dilutions equal amounts of a 2 per cent sheep erythrocytes suspension and incubate in water bath at 37° C for 15 min; the "hemolytic system" is ready.

Distribute 0.20 ml of each hemolysin dilution-sheep erythrocytes mixture to each vertical row of (a) set of tubes, starting from the next to last to the right and using the same pipette to the lowest dilution. In the ninth vertical row 0.20 ml of vbs is distributed, instead of the hemolysin dilution, as complement control.

Dilute furthermore a $1/30$ dilution of complement as follows:

Complement 1/30	ml	0.3	0.3	0.3	0.3	0.3	0.3	0.3
Veronal b s	ml	0.1	0.2	0.3	0.4	0.5	0.6	0.7
Final dilutions		1/40	1/50	1/60	1/70	1/80	1/90	1/100

Distribute 0.20 ml of each complement dilution in each horizon-

---

* Veronal buffer solution: NaCl 85.0 gm

  5-5 diethylbarbituric acid 5.75 gm

  5-5 sodic diethylbarbiturate 3.75 gm

Dissolve diethylbarbituric acid in boiling distilled H_2O, then add the other constituents and distilled H_2O up to 2.0 liter.

Add:

  $MgCl_2$ • $6H_2O$ 1.68 gm

  $CaCl_2$ dry 0.28 gm

Autoclave at ½ atmosphere for 20 min. Solution has a 7.2 pH. Store at 4° C and dilute to ⅕ when used. Discard unused ⅕ dilution.

tal row, starting from the next to last and using the same pipette to the lowest dilution.

Distribute in the last row, 0.20 ml of vbs as hemolysin control.

Place in one tube only the erythrocytes suspension and vbs to reach the standard volume as erythrocytes control.

Shake well and incubate at 37° C for 45 min in the water bath.

Read for results.

Titration

One Hemolytic Unit (HU) is contained in the highest dilution of hemolysin and complement where complete hemolysis is obtained.

Complement titration

Dilute complement as described above.

Distribute 0.20 ml of complement dilutions in seven serology tubes.

Add 0.40 ml of vbs to replace antigen and serum.

Add 0.20 ml of the hemolytic system, prepared as described above, containing 4 HU.

Incubate in water bath at 37° C for 45 min.

Read for results.

Titration

One unit of complement is contained in the highest dilution of complement where complete hemolysis is obtained.

Antigen titration

Set up eight horizontal rows with eight serology tubes each.

Distribute 0.20 ml of undiluted antigen in seven tubes of the first vertical row, and 0.20 ml of antigen diluted ½, ¼, ⅛, ... ¹⁄₆₄, respectively, in the seven tubes of the second, third, ... seventh vertical row, beginning from the right with the highest dilution and using the same pipette. In the eighth vertical row, distribute 0.20 ml of vbs as antiserum control.

Dilute known, inactivated, positive antiserum ¼, ⅛, ¹⁄₁₆, ... ¹⁄₆₄, or more, and distribute 0.20 ml of each dilution, respectively, in each horizontal row, beginning from the bottom with the highest dilution and using the same pipette.

Distribute 0.20 ml of vbs in the last row as antigen control.

Distribute 0.20 ml of complement, containing 2 units, in all tubes.

Prepare, in a further horizontal row, controls for complement and hemolytic system:

  (a) Distribute 0.40 ml of vbs in four tubes to replace the volumes of antigen and antiserum. To the first tube to the left add 0.20 ml of complement, as used in titration, containing 2 units; to the second, third and fourth, add 0.20 ml of complement diluted to contain 1, ½, ¼ units of complement respectively.

  (b) Distribute 0.60 ml of vbs to one tube to replace the volumes of antigen, antiserum, and complement.

Add 0.20 ml of the hemolytic system, prepared as described above, to all the tubes.

Incubate in water bath at 37° C for 45 min.

Read for results.

Titration

One unit of antigen is contained in the highest dilution of antigen combined with the highest dilution of serum in which complement-fixation occurs (where hemolysis is obtained).

Antibody titration (Complement-fixation test)

Dilute inactivated serum to be tested ¼, ⅛, ¹⁄₁₆, ... ¹⁄₂₅₆ in vbs.

Set up one horizontal row of ten tubes for each antigen used.

Distribute 0.20 ml of the ¹⁄₂₅₆ serum dilution to the seventh tube on the right, and the same volume of the succeeding decreasing dilutions in the sixth, fifth, ... first tube, using the same pipette.

Distribute 0.20 ml of an antigen dilution containing 2 units to each tube.

Prepare controls as follows:

  (a) For serum control: distribute 0.20 ml of serum diluted ¼, ⅛, ¹⁄₁₆ in three separate tubes and add to each one 0.20 ml of vbs to replace the antigen.

(b) For antigen control: distribute 0.20 ml of the antigen dilution used in the test in two tubes, and 0.20 ml of vbs to replace serum.

(c) For antigen activity control: challenge the antigen with a known specific antiserum, as described for the unknown serum to be tested.

(d) For complement control: as described in (a) of antigen titration paragraph.

(e) For hemolytic system control: distribute 0.60 ml of vbs in tubes to replace serum, complement, and antigen. (See note.)

Distribute 0.20 ml of a dilution containing 2 units of complement in all tubes (for complement control: 2, 1, ½, ¼ units).

Store at 4° C for 18 hr.

Add 0.20 ml of the hemolytic system, prepared as described above, to all tubes, containing 4 to 8 HU.

Incubate in water bath at 37° C for 45 min.

Read for results.

Interpretation of the results

Hemolysis must occur in all control tubes except:

(a) in the hemolytic system control;

(b) in the last two tubes (containing ½ and ¼ units) of complement control, and

(c) in some or all the antigen activity control tubes, depending on the titer.

The positivity of the test is given by the absence of hemolysis and is indicated as 1, 2, 3, 4 + when the 25, 50, 75, 100 per cent of hemolysis is estimated.

Note: It is very useful to set up controls for possible antibodies in the serum towards the tissue cultures, the chick tissues or fluids, and the animal tissues used in the cultivation of viruses.

Modifications to the complement-fixation test method

In order to reduce the amount of expensive viral antigens to be used in C-F tests and to make the test itself less time-consuming when dealing with many sera and antigens, some modifications have been introduced to C-F test standard technique.

C-F test on perspex sheets [30]

This test is carried on square perspex sheets of various dimensions, generally 12 x 12 x ¼ in. Every sheet is marked off in 100 squares of about 1 in per side. Letters and numbers of reference for vertical and horizontal columns and rows are impressed on the sides. The preparation of the constituents of the reaction is much the same as described for the standard method: 0.02 ml of each reagent are placed on the center of the squares by means of tuberculin syringes in which N° 19 hypodermic needles (with the beveled tips cut out) are fitted.

The arrangement of the dilutions, controls, etc. is similar to the one employed with the standard method.

The sheet, or the sheets, are then placed on a rack and the rack is placed into a metal air-tight box containing a layer of cotton soaked with water.

After 18 hr at 4° C, 0.02 ml of the hemolytic system are added to each test square and the rack is again placed into the box and incubated at 37° C for 30 min.

After incubation, each test square is observed for hemolysis. The reading of the results is similar to that described for the standard method.

Rapid microtechnique C-F test [29]

This test, employing the rapid microtechnique, is carried out on plastic plates each having 96 cylindrical cells 6 mm in diameter.

For the dilution and distribution procedures, spiral loops of 0.025 ml capacity are used. This method brings down to about ⅛ the amount of reagents to be employed compared to the standard method.

Complement-fixation test (Indirect method) [2]

Sometimes birds infected with psittacosis virus fail to produce antibodies which usually can be detected by the complement-fixation techinque.

In these cases an indirect method is used, namely a neutralization test in which the C-F test is used as an indicator.

3. NEUTRALIZATION TEST [10, 15, 17]

The neutralization test is performed on animals, embryonated eggs, or cell cultures, according to the ability of the particular virus to reproduce in one or the other medium.

The route of inoculation for the animals and eggs depends on the characteristics of the agent.

When it is possible to use them, tissue cultures are preferred because they are easier to handle and much more uniform in the results.

When embryonated eggs are used, it must be taken into account that three different end points for titration can be used as follows: (a) variations in the death of embryos; (b) variations in the number of visible lesions on the chorionallantoic membrane, and (c) when dealing with hemagglutinins producing viruses, the variation in hemagglutinin production.

In neutralization tests, both the virus suspension and the serum dilutions may vary. The serum dilutions are commonly used in diagnostic work as very slight changes in antibodies titers can be detected better, even when low titer antigens are employed.

Virus titration

Prepare 0.5 $\log_{10}$ ($\frac{1}{10}$, $\frac{1}{32}$, $\frac{1}{100}$, $\frac{1}{320}$, $\frac{1}{1000}$, $\frac{1}{3,200}$) dilutions of the virus suspension in an ice bath, using different pipettes for each dilution; sterile saline containing 0.5 per cent of bovine albumin should be used for diluting if animals or chick embryos are to be inoculated. If tissue cultures are used, the dilutions will be carried on the same solution used for cell maintenance.

Inoculate six animals or eggs per dilution, with a sufficient amount of virus suspension to produce infection, at least with the lowest dilutions. When using tissue cultures, 0.10 ml of each dilution is inoculated respectively in six tubes.

Incubate eggs and tissue cultures at proper temperature, which may vary for some viruses.

Daily observation will be maintained on the animals and eggs and microscopic readings of the tissue cultures taken until the effect of the inoculation is noticed. This lapse of time may vary remarkably, depending on the type of virus used. The titration is not reliable if more than half of the animals or embryos die or if some deaths occur within 24 hr of the inoculation, presumably for traumatic reasons.

The infectious (ID), or lethal (LD), or cytopathic (TCD) dose 100 per cent is the highest dilution of the virus which causes infection, death, or generalized cytopathic degeneration of the animals, eggs, or tissue cultures.

The 50 per cent end points (ID_{50}, LD_{50}, TCD_{50}) are calculated according to the Reed and Muench or Kärber methods.

Antibody titration (Neutralization test) [18]

Prepare 0.5 $\log_{10}$ dilutions of the serum to be tested, using the same diluents indicated for the virus titration and changing pipettes for each dilution.

Mix equal volumes of the serum dilutions and the virus suspension so that the final mixture contains 100 D_{50}/inoculum and incubate at 37° C for one or more hours, depending on the type of virus used. Sometimes it is convenient to prolong the time of contact, as for polio viruses, up to 6 hr at 37° C and then at 4° C for 18 hr.

Inoculate four to six animals, embryonated eggs, or tissue culture tubes per dilution with a volume of the serum dilution-virus suspension mixture containing 100 D_{50} (usually 100 TCD_{50}/ 0.10 ml for tissue cultures).

Prepare the following controls:

(a) uninoculated animals, embryos, or tissue cultures, for nonspecific infection or degeneration;

(b) titration of the virus with the same concentration used in the test and diluted 10^{-1}, 10^{-2}, 10^{-3}, for virus activity;

(c) inoculate serum in controls at the lowest dilution used in the test for toxicity, and

(d) challenge known positive antiserum with virus for reference titer and purity of the strain.

Interpretation of the results

After periods of observations, varying in length due to the characteristics of the virus employed, results are recorded. A point of reference for the observation time are the controls, inoculated with the standard suspension of virus alone.

No changes should appear in controls (a) and (c) and in about 50 per cent of the 10^{-2} and 10^{-3} dilutions of (b).

Changes will appear in (d) according to the titer of the known antiserum.

The neutralization titer of the serum is calculated following the Reed and Muench or the Kärber methods. An increase in neutralization titer, in the course of the disease, is of diagnostic significance.

Modifications to the Neutralization Standard Method in Tissue Cultures

(a) *Rapid microscopic method* [19]

Sterilized, flat-bottom tubes are used in this test and a reversed microscope is necessary for the observations.

Titration of virus

Dilute virus suspension as described for the standard method. (See page 67).

Distribute 0.4 ml of virus suspension in six tubes for each dilution.

Add 0.10 ml of the bs used in diluting virus suspension to all tubes to replace serum.

Prepare a rich cell suspension (2×10^5 for monkey kidney cells) in a double concentrated medium.

Add 0.5 ml of cell suspension to each virus dilution tube.

Add 0.4 ml of sterilized vaseline oil to each tube.

Incubate open tubes at 37° C for four to eight days in a vertical position.

Calculate the $TCID_{50}$ according to the Reed and Muench or Kärber method.

Neutralization test

Dilute inactivated serum (56° C for 30 min) as described for the standard method.

Distribute 0.1 ml of each serum dilution in six separate tubes.

Prepare the same controls as in standard methods.

Distribute 0.4 ml of virus suspension diluted to contain 100 $TCID_{50}$ in all tubes containing serum dilutions and in the proper control tubes.

Add 0.5 ml of cell suspension prepared as described for virus titration to all tubes.

Add 0.4 ml of sterile vaseline oil and incubate as described above; observation time may vary from four to eight days.

Interpretation of the results

The neutralization titer of serum is calculated according to the Reed and Muench or Kärber methods on the basis of the number of cultures unprotected from virus cytopathic effect.

(b) *Immunoinactivation method* [20]

This method is used only with some viruses, such as polio viruses and Theiler's virus, and is different from the standard method only in the time of contact between serum dilutions and virus suspension.

Higher titers are observed in this way.

Serum dilutions begin from $1/10$ and the time of contact is 6 hr at 37° C, followed by 12 hr at 4° C.

(c) *Neutralization Test in Agar Cultures* [5, 11, 20]

For the preparation of agar cell cultures, we refer to the various methods commonly used.

Technique of the test

Discard the nutrient medium and wash the cell layer three times with phosphate buffer solution (pbs).[†]

---

† Phosphate Buffer Solution (pbs):

Add 0.2 ml of an equal mixture of two-fold serum dilutions and virus suspension containing 1.000 PFU/ml (Plaque Forming Unit) to each tissue culture (two or more tissue cultures per dilution).

Incubate at 37° C for 1 hr (for polio viruses see b).

After incubation, add the melted agar according to the method of choice.

Read for results after three to six days of incubation.

Interpretation of the results

The titer is given by the dilution of serum which inhibits 95 to 100 per cent of 100 PFU inoculated.

(d) *pH Color Test (Salk Test)* [12, 25]

This test is based on the fact that, in tissue cultures, cells acidify the medium for their own metabolic activity. Thus the phenol red contained in the medium turns gradually from red at pH 7.4 to 7.8 to salmon at 7.2 and finally to various degrees of yellow, below 6.9.

If a cytopathic virus is added to a tissue culture, the cell metabolism is altered in some way and thus the changes in color

Solution A	
KCl	2.0 gm
KH_2PO_4	2.0 gm
$Na_2HPO_4 \cdot 2H_2O$	14.4 gm
NaCl	80.0 gm
H_2O (bidistilled)	800.0 ml
Solution B	
$CaCl_2$	0.5 gm
H_2O (bidistilled)	500.0 ml
Solution C	
$MgCl_2 \cdot 6H_2O$	0.5 gm
H_2O (bidistilled)	500.0 ml

Autoclave at 0.6 atmosphere for 10 min.

Mix:

H_2O (sterile, bidistilled)	720.0 ml
Solution A	80.0 ml
Solution B	100.0 ml
Solution C	100.0 ml

of the medium are different from those in the control noninoculated cultures.

Titration of virus

Centrifuge at 500 rpm for 1 min trypsinized cells.

Resuspend in nutrient medium (i.e., S.M. 199 95 per cent; horse serum 2 per cent; sodium bicarbonate (2.8 per cent) 3 per cent; penicillin 200 UI/ml; streptomycin mg 0.1/ml) to a concentration of 3 x 10^5 cells/ml.‡

Sterilize plastic dishes by rinsing thoroughly in tap water, bidistilled H$_2$O, and eventually in 70 per cent alcohol. Ultraviolet light can be added to the sterilization process.

Distribute in four wells/dilution 1.0 ml of nutrient medium, 0.5 ml of the virus 0.5 log$_{10}$ dilutions in Hanks, and 0.5 ml of the cell suspension. To distribute uniformly the various components, a Cornwall continuous pipetting unit is commonly used.

Prepare the following controls:

(a) Uninoculated cells, for normal metabolism of cells; replace virus inoculum with 0.5 ml of Hanks.

(b) Prepare a complete system free of cells, for the stability of the medium and for the effect of virus suspension on it.

Seal wells with sterile paraffin oil.

Place a sheet of sterilized aluminum foil over the dishes as covering and incubate at 37° C for some days.

Read for the changes in color and record the results.

Some authors suggest the addition, two days before the final reading, of 1 drop of a 10 per cent glucose solution in bidistilled H$_2$O to each well for a better differentiation of positive and negative cultures.

---

‡ Cell count: Prepare a 1 per cent solution in citric acid 0.1M (19.212 gm in 1,000 ml of distilled H$_2$O) of crystal violet.

Mix 1.0 ml of cell suspension with 1 drop of dye diluted 1/10.

Place 1 drop of the cell suspension-dye mixture on a Thoma hemocytometer and count cells on the total area.

Repeat the count three times, make an average of results, and multiply by 10,000 to obtain cell concentration/cubic ml.

Interpretation of the results

Where the color appears unchanged, growth of virus has been obtained. Control wells and those containing cells not under cytopathic effect will turn yellow.

The $TCID_{50}$ is calculated according to the Reed and Muench or Kärber method.

Antibody Titration (Neutralization Test)

Inactivate serum to be tested at 56° C for 30 min.

Mix 0.25 ml of two-fold dilutions of serum in Hanks, with 0.50 ml of a virus-cell suspension mixture (0.25 ml + 0.25 ml) containing 100 $TCID_{50}$.

Distribute as described for the titration of the virus, employing four to six wells for each serum dilution.

Prepare the following controls:

(a) Virus suspension containing 100 $TCID_{50}$, as used in the test, and diluted 10^{-1}, 10^{-2}, 10^{-3}, for virus activity;

(b) Repeat test using a known positive antiserum, for reference titer;

(c) Inoculate serum and replace virus suspension, for excluding any toxic effect of serum on cells, and

(d) Uninoculated cells, for nonspecific infection or degeneration and for color comparison.

Incubate at 37° C for some days after sealing wells and dishes as described above.

Interpretation of the results

As described above, protection from cytopathic effect by the serum is revealed by a color behavior similar among inoculated cells and (d) controls.

The neutralization titer of the serum is calculated according to the Reed and Muench or Kärber method.

4. HEMAGGLUTINATION-INHIBITION TEST [23]

The hemagglutinating ability of some viruses (mumps, Newcastle, dengue, yellow fever, encephalitis, etc.) is neutralized (inhibited) by the specific antibodies. The test is, *per se*, very simple to perform, but the strain specificity (i.e., in influenza) and the presence of nonspecific inhibitors in human sera limit in some way the reliability of its applications.

Hemagglutinating antigen titration

Distribute 0.25 ml of two-fold dilutions of antigen in buffered saline (bs) at pH 7.1 to 7.2, beginning from ½ to $\frac{1}{1,024}$ in serology tubes or in eighty-wells Perspex dishes.

Add 0.25 ml of bs to all the tubes or wells.

Add 0.50 ml of 0.5 per cent erythrocytes suspension (human, fowl, etc.) and shake gently.

Prepare a control by mixing 0.5 ml of bs to 0.5 ml of erythrocytes suspension for autoagglutination.

Keep at room temperature (4° C for influenza virus C) for 45 to 60 min.

Read for results.

Interpretation of the results

The highest dilution of antigen in which agglutination of erythrocytes is observed contains 1 hemagglutinating unit (HA unit).

Antibody titration (Hemagglutination-Inhibition Test)

Serum:

Inactivate serum at 56° C for 30 min.

In order to eliminate any nonspecific inhibitors which may be present in the serum, mix 1.0 ml of potassium periodate 0.015/M solution, freshly prepared, with 0.5 ml of serum.

Keep at 4° C for 18 hr.

Add 1.0 ml of 1 per cent glycerol solution in bs.

At this stage, the serum is diluted ⅕.

Technique of the test

Distribute 0.25 ml of bs starting from the second tube, or well if using a Perspex dish.

Distribute 0.25 ml of the ⅕ serum dilution to the first and second tube or well.

Pass 0.25 ml of the serum dilution from the second to the third tube or well, from the third to the fourth, and so on to the highest dilution, discarding 0.25 ml from the last.

Add 0.25 ml of antigen dilution containing 8 HA units to all tubes or wells.

Add 0.5 ml of a 0.5 per cent suspension of erythrocytes to all tubes or wells.

Prepare the following controls:

(a) Set up a separate hemagglutination test using the standard dilution of antigen and ½, ¼, ⅛, ¹⁄₁₆ dilutions of the standard for HA unit control.

(b) Add 0.5 ml of 0.5 per cent erythrocytes suspension to 0.5 ml of bs for incidental autoagglutination of erythrocytes;

(c) Add to 0.25 ml of serum (⅕), 0.25 ml of bs, and 0.5 ml of 0.5 per cent erythrocytes suspension, for incidental agglutination power of the serum;

(d) Set up a test with a known specific antiserum, for reference titer, and

(e) Repeat as in (c) for incidental agglutinating power of known antiserum.

Keep at room temperature (4° C for influenza virus C) for 45 to 60 min.

Read for results.

Interpretation of the test

The titer of the serum is given by the highest dilution in which a complete inhibition of hemolysis is observed.

Note: Preparation of bs (pH 7.1-7.2):

NaCl	8.5 g
H_2O dist.	200.0 ml
Add:	
$NaHPO_4$ (0.5/M) solution	13.8 ml
$NaH_2PO_4 \cdot H_2O$ (0.5/M) solution	6.2 ml
Add:	
H_2O dist. up to	1.000 ml

Note: The following technique can also be employed for treating serum:

Inactivate serum at 56° C for 30 min.

Trypsinize serum by mixing 1 volume of it with ½ volume of 0.8 per cent trypsin solution in 0.1 M phosphate buffer (pH 8.2).

Incubate at 56° C for 30 min.

Mix 1 volume of trypsin treated serum with 3 volumes M/90 aqueous periodate.

Incubate at room temperature for 15 min.

Add 1 volume of 1 per cent glycerin in saline.

Incubate at room temperature for 15 min.

The various passages dilute serum ⅐; bring it to 1/10 before use.

When dealing with encephalitis viruses the technique employed for treating serum is as follows:

Inactivate serum at 56° C for 30 min.

Mix 1 volume of serum with 4 volumes of saline (pH 9.0) and 5 volumes of 25 per cent kaolin (pH 9.0).

Incubate at room temperature, shaking frequently.

Centrifuge at 2,500 rpm for 30 min.

Recuperate serum which is now diluted 1/10.

5. ARBOVIRUSES CLASSIFICATION

The number of known arboviruses has enormously increased in the last few years. Among the complement-fixation tests, the neutralization and the hemagglutino-inhibition tests, the latter seems to be the more reliable.

In the following table the classification of the arboviruses is given.

ARBOVIRUSES CLASSIFICATION

According to W H O Technical Report Series 1961, No. 219

Group A: Aura (BeAr 10315)
Chikungunya
E E E
O'nyong-nyong
Mayaro
Middelburg
Semliki
Sindbis
Una   (BeAr 13136)
Uruna
V E E
W E E

AMM 2021
Sagiyama   } Identical?
AMM 2354

Group B: Bat salivary gland (Rio Brava)
Bussuquara
Dengue type I°
Dengue type II°
Dengue type III°
Dengue type IV°
Ilheus
Japanese B
Modoc
M V encephalitis
Ntaya
Spondweny
St Louis
Turkey meningoencephalitis
Uganda S
Wesselbron
West Nile
Yellow fever
Zika
AMM 1775
SA H 336 (similar to Uganda S)
Diphasic meningoencephalitis
Central European tick or milk-borne encephalitis
Kyasanur forest disease
Langat (TP 21)
Louping Ill
Omsk haemorragic fever
Powassan
Russian spring-summer encephalitis

Group C: Apeu (An 848)
Caraparu (An 3994)
Marituba (An 15)
Murutucu (An 974)
Oriboca (An 17)
Itaqui (An 12797)

Bunyamwera group: Bunyamwera
Cache Valley
Chittoor
Germiston
Guaroa
Ilesha
Kairi
Weyomyia

Other groups: I°   California encephalitis
Trivittatus   (This group may be part of the
Melao   Bunyamwera group.)
Be Ar 8033

                II°   Guama
Catu
Bimiti

                III°   Bwamba
Pongola

IV°   Simbu
        Oropouche
        Sathuperi

V°   Turlock
        Umbre

VI°   Anopheles A
        Anopheles B
        TR 10076

VII°   AMM 2549
        AMM 2325

VIII°   Tr 7994
        Tr 8762
        Tr 9223

IX°   Quaranfil
        Chenuda
        Eg Ar 1306

Ungrouped: African horse sickness
                            Blue tongue
                            Colorado tick fever
                            Crimean haemorragic fever
                            Nairobi sheep disease
                            Sandfly fever, Neapolitan strain
                            Sandfly fever, Sicilian strain
                            Hart Park
                            Manganilla (Tr 3587)
                            Rift Valley fever
                            Tacaiuma (Be An 73)
                            Witwatersrand (Sa Ar 1062)
                            Argentinian haemorragic fever (Junin virus)

6. HEMABSORPTION-INHIBITION TEST [21]

Tissue cultures inoculated with viruses of the influenza and parainfluenza groups acquire the property of fixing chicken and guinea pigs erythrocytes on the cell surface.

Sera containing specific antibodies neutralize (inhibit) such capacity.

Technique of the test

(a) Inoculate ten to twelve tissue culture tubes, for each serum to be tested, with an hemabsorbing virus.

Incubate at 37° C for three days.

Check the degree of hemabsorption in one or two of the tubes by adding 0.2 ml of chicken or guinea pig washed erythrocytes 0.5 per cent suspension in bs to each tube and incubating at 4° C for 20 min.

Repeat as above until a high degree of positivity is observed.

(b) Prepare two-fold serum dilutions in Hanks solution, starting from $\frac{1}{8}$ to $\frac{1}{1,024}$.

Discard the maintenance solutions from the tissue culture tubes and wash the cells twice with 1.0 ml of Hanks solution.

Add 1.0 ml of serum dilutions to tissue cultures, using two tubes for each dilution so that the cells result completely covered when the tubes are horizontal.

Keep at room temperature for 20 min.

Add 0.20 ml of a 0.5 per cent erythrocytes suspension, as described above.

Incubate at 4° C for 20 min.

Prepare the following controls:

(a) Uninoculated cells, for spontaneous hemabsorption;

(b) Known specific antiserum, for reference titer;

(c) Unchallenged virus, for hemabsorption activity.

Read for results.

Interpretation of the results

Serum titer is given by the highest dilution able to inhibit completely hemabsorption as observed microscopically.

The following technique may also be used for Hemabsorption-inhibition test:

Prepare two-fold dilutions of inactivated serum in Hanks solution.

Mix 0.2 ml of each serum dilution with 0.2 ml of virus suspension, containing 100 $TCID_{50}/0.1$ ml.

Incubate at room temperature for 1 hr and inoculate two tissue culture tubes for each serum dilution-virus suspension mixture.

Incubate at 36° C.

After six days add 0.2 ml of a 0.4 per cent guinea pig erythrocytes suspension.

Incubate at 4° C for 30 min.

Prepare the same controls as above.

Read for results.

Interpretation of the results

As above.

7. COLD HEMAGGLUTINATION TEST [6, 8]

This test is used as an aid in the diagnosis of primary atypical pneumonia. It is not specific and the results are affected by various factors, such as the severity and duration of the illness, the level of the febrile reaction, etc.

Cold hemagglutinins generally appear around the second week of the disease.

Technique of the test [3,27]

Serum: Once drawn, the blood should be kept at room temperature, and not in the refrigerator, to avoid the removal by homologous erythrocytes of hemagglutinins from the serum.

As in some high titer sera, hemagglutinins may absorb on cells at room temperature also; it is useful to warm the blood sample to 37° C before separating serum.

The serum can be kept frozen at −20° C for a number of years without any significant decrease of titer. At 4° C, however, the loss is appreciable, and at room temperature may be rather fast.

Serum can be used after inactivation.

Erythrocytes: Human erythrocytes of the O-group, from two to four days old, are used for the test.

Wash erythrocytes in saline and centrifuge at 1,000 rpm for 10 min; discard the supernatant.

Repeat such washing procedure three times.

Eventually, discard the supernatant and centrigue again in saline in a graduated tube at 1,500 rpm for 15 min. Calculate the volume of the packed cells.

Suspend the packed erythrocytes in saline to make a 0.2 per cent suspension.

Technique of the test

Prepare two-fold dilutions of serum in saline and distribute 0.5 ml of each dilution in separate tubes.

Add 0.5 ml of the 0.2 per cent suspension of erythrocytes; the final dilutions are now doubled.

Prepare the following controls:

(a) add 0.5 ml of saline to 0.5 ml of erythrocytes suspension, for autoagglutination control, and

(b) repeat test with known positive antiserum, for reference titer and agglutinability of erythrocytes.

Incubate at 4° C for about 12 hr.

Read immediately after taking out of cold room.

After reading, store at 37° C for 30 min, again, to make agglutination disappear in positive tubes and to control the absence of heteroagglutination or of other antibodies which may be responsible for hemagglutination.

Interpretation of the results

The maximum of positivity (indicated as 4+) is considered reached when the cells are all agglutinated and do not become free on gentle shaking of the tubes.

The end point is taken on the minimal agglutination at the highest dilution.

In primary atypical pneumonia, titers may reach $\frac{1}{1,080}$ or more. It is more significant, for diagnostic purposes, to observe an increase (four-fold) in the titer during the course of the disease, rather than a single, high titer.

Cold hemagglutinins have been observed and studied in many diseases. Though their presence or absence do not definitely demonstrate or exclude a primary atypical pneumonia, only in this infection do single titers and the increase of values seem to be so high.

8. STREPTOCOCCUS MG AGGLUTINATION TEST

This test is used as an aid in retrospective diagnosis of primary atypical pneumonia, as agglutinins usually reach their maximum titer from four to five weeks after the onset of the disease.

The test is not specific and is not necessarily correlated to cold hemagglutinins.

The results are affected by the various factors described for cold hemagglutination.[31, 32]

Serum

Inactivate serum at 56° C for 30 min.

Preparation of the antigen[28]

Inoculate 200.0 ml of trypticase soy broth with 0.2 ml of an 18 hr
    broth culture of Streptococcus MG.
Incubate at 37° C for 18 hr.
Centrifuge at 1,500 rpm for 30 min and discard the supernatant.
Wash and centrifuge three times in sterile saline.
Discard the third washing supernatant and heat at 56° C for 2
    hr, shaking frequently.
Set up a sterility test by inoculating one loopful of the microbic
    bulk in trypticase soy broth.
If sterile, the antigen is stored at 4° C up to several months.
When used, dilute in sterile saline to a turbidity of tube N° 3
    of McFarland nephelometer.
Check the diluted antigen and, from time to time, the stored
    antigen for a positive Quellung test and for agglutination with
    known rabbit Streptococcus MG antiserum.

Technique of the test

Prepare serial two-fold dilutions, in saline, of inactivated serum
    and distribute 0.5 ml in separate serology tubes.
Add 0.5 ml of diluted antigen to each tube; the final serum dilu-
    tions are now doubled.
Prepare the following controls:

(a) add 0.5 ml of saline to 0.5 ml of antigen, for autoagglu-
    tination control, and
(b) prepare an agglutination test using known positive anti-
    serum for reference titer and agglutinability of the an-
    tigen.

Shake the tubes well and incubate at 37° C for 2 hr and then at
    4° C for about 12 hr.
Read for results.

Interpretation of the results

The same considerations made for the cold agglutination test
can be applied to the Streptococcus MG agglutination.

9. MACACUS RHESUS ERYTHROCYTES AGGLUTINATION TEST [9, 13] (Hoyt-Morrison Test)

The Hoyt-Morrison test is today widely employed in infectious hepatitis (ih) diagnostic.

It is not a specific test and agglutination is probably due to some factors forming in the patient's sera in the course of illness.

The test is positive in about 86 per cent of acute cases of ih, but sometimes positive agglutinations may be observed in the course of other diseases.

Preparation of the materials for the test

Serum: Sterilely drawn and inactivated at 56° C for 30 min.

M. rhesus erythrocytes: Freshly and sterilely drawn, washed several times in ps and resuspended in ps to a 2 per cent concentration.

Technique of the test

Prepare a two-fold dilution in ps of inactivated serum, beginning from ½ up to 1/320, or over.

Distribute 0.2 ml of each dilution in separate serology tubes.

Prepare the following controls:

(a) replace serum with ps in one tube, for autoagglutination control, and

(b) use a ⅛ dilution of known positive serum, for erythrocytes agglutinability control.

Add to each tube 0.2 ml of M. rhesus erythrocytes suspension.

Incubate in water bath at 37° C for 1 hr.

Centrifuge at 500 rpm for 2 min.

Shake tubes gently under a proper light.

Read for results.

Interpretation of the test

Significant titers start from ⅛.

In acute cases, as mentioned above, the positivity is about 86 per cent, while in chronic cases it decreases to about 71 per cent. Such positivity may disappear after a rather short time or it may be present for approximately three years after infection.

10. INFECTIOUS MONONUCLEOSIS

During the course of the disease, heterophile antibodies are produced. These antibodies agglutinate sheep erythrocytes and are not specific of the disease, as they can be found in a number of normal sera and in the sera of vaccinated individuals.

It is possible, however, to distinguish among these different antibodies through differential absorptions on guinea pig kidney and beef erythrocytes.[26]

The following scheme shows the behavior of sera unabsorbed or after absorption.

Normal serum:

Unabsorbed: may or may not agglutinate sheep erythrocytes.
Absorbed on guinea pig kidney: does not agglutinate sheep erythrocytes.
Absorbed on beef erythrocytes: behaves like unabsorbed serum.

Serum from individual after serum therapy:

Unabsorbed: agglutinates sheep erythrocytes.
Absorbed on guinea pig kidney: does not agglutinate sheep erythrocytes.
Absorbed on beef erythrocytes: does not agglutinate sheep erythrocytes.

Serum from infectious mononucleosis case:

Unabsorbed: agglutinates sheep erythrocytes.
Absorbed on guinea pig kidney: agglutinates sheep erythrocytes.
Absorbed on beef erythrocytes: does not agglutinate sheep erythrocytes.

Agglutination Test (Paul-Bunnel-Davidsohn Test) [14]

Preparation of the antigen

Defibrinate sterile sheep blood by shaking in a glass container with glass beads.

Centrifuge 4 to 5.0 ml of defibrinated blood at 1,500 rpm for 10 min.

Discard the supernatant and wash three times with 10.0 ml of sterile ps; centrifuge after each washing.

If, after discarding, the last washing fluid is clear and colorless, add 99.0 ml of ps to 1.0 ml of erythrocytes suspension.

Store at 4° C up to about one week (antigen should not be used if any hemolysis appears).

Serum

Inactivate serum at 56° C for 30 min in water bath.

Technique of the test

Prepare a two-fold dilution in sterile ps of serum to be tested, beginning from $\frac{1}{5}$ to $\frac{1}{640}$.

Distribute 0.5 ml of each dilution in eight separate serology tubes.

Place 0.5 ml of sterile ps into one tube, for autoagglutination control.

Add, after gentle shaking of the container, 0.5 ml of the erythrocytes suspension to each tube; the final serum dilutions range now from $\frac{1}{10}$ to $\frac{1}{1,280}$.

Shake well and incubate at 37° C for 2 hr.

Incubate at 4° C for about 12 hr.

Read for results.

Absorption of serum with guinea pig kidney

Mince fresh guinea pig kidney and grind in a sterile porcelain mortar.

Rub the ground kidney through a piece of cloth.

Add 15.0 ml of distilled H_2O and centrifuge at 3,000 rpm for 20 min.

Repeat washing and centrifuging operations three more times.

Discard the last supernatant and suspend the sediment to 20 per cent concentration in sterile ps. Store at −20° C until used.

Mix 1.0 ml of guinea pig kidney suspension with 1.0 ml of 1/2.5 dilution of inactivated serum to be tested.

Incubate at 37° C for 30 min in water bath.

Centrifuge at 4,000 rpm for 20 min.

Recuperate the supernatant, which is the absorbed serum diluted $\frac{1}{5}$.

Technique of the test

It is similar in all details to the technique described above.

Interpretation of the results

A positive agglutination is strongly indicative for infectious mononucleosis. The comparison between unabsorbed and absorbed serum from the same patient will give the extent of absorption of heterophile antibodies by guinea pig kidney.

11. RICKETTSIA

Serological Tests and Their Interpretation in Rickettsial Infections[7]

(a) Louse and flea-borne rickettsial infections.

Rickettsia mooseri (Murine typhus)

Agglutinins for Proteus OX 19 appear between the sixth and the eighth days of illness, showing a titer of about $\frac{1}{200}$. During the following days the titer will usually rise to $\frac{1}{1,000}$.

At the same time agglutinins for R. mooseri appear and the highest titer may reach $\frac{1}{5,000}$ at the end of the second week. This titer level remains unmodified for about two months and the decrease is progressive, taking one year, more or less.

Complement-fixing antibodies appear between the tenth and the twentieth days of illness. At the end of the first month the titer may reach $\frac{1}{640}$.

Rickettsia prowazeki (Epidemic typhus)

Agglutinins for Proteus OX 19 first appear about the fifth day of illness and are detectable for about two months after recovery.

Titers may reach values of over $\frac{1}{6,400}$ during the second week.

Agglutinins for R. prowazeki are present, but the results of the agglutination test may not be uniform.

Between the fifth and the tenth days, the complement-fixing antibodies will appear and titers may be as high as $\frac{1}{1,000}$.

Brill's disease

Agglutination for Proteus OX 19 is usually negative.

Agglutination for R. prowazeki and complement-fixation tests are helpful in diagnosing the disease.

Rickettsia quintana (Trench fever)

Agglutinations for Proteus OX 2, OX 19, and OX K are negative.

Agglutinins and complement-fixing antibodies for R. quintana are demonstrable, but the specific antigens are difficult to prepare as the rickettsia does not infect embryonated eggs or small animals.

(b) Tick-borne rickettsial infections

Rickettsia australis (North Queensland tick typhus)

Agglutinins for Proteus OX 19, at low titers, can be observed. At lower titers, still, for OX 2.

The best choice is the complement-fixation test.

Rickettsia brasiliensis (São Paulo typhus)

Agglutination for the three strains of Proteus can be observed at low titers.

Rickettsia conori (Fiévre boutonneuse)

Agglutinins for Proteus OX 2 and OX 19 appear at about the tenth day of illness at medium titers; from $\frac{1}{50}$ to $\frac{1}{500}$. If Proteus OX 2 is agglutinated at higher titers than OX 19, or is agglutinated alone, it will probably be due to a R. conori infection.

The complement-fixation test is specific and permits, when an increase of C-F antibodies is observed in the course of the disease, the definition of its etiology.

Rickettsia rickettsi (Spotted fever)

Agglutinins for Proteus OX 2 and OX 19 appear about the

sixth day of illness. The highest titer is reached about the twelfth day and is significant when over $\frac{1}{320}$ or when an increase is observed in the course of the disease.

The titer for one of the two types is usually higher. Agglutinins for R. rickettsi appear about the same time and titers may reach very high values.

The complement-fixation test is specific with "washed" antigens.

Rickettsia rickettsi var pijperi (South African tick-bite fever)

Agglutinins for Proteus OX 2 and OX 19 appear about the eleventh day of illness. The highest titers ($\frac{1}{3,200}$) are reached about the third week.

Proteus OX 2 is usually agglutinated at higher dilutions. Low titers for Proteus OX K may sometimes be observed.

The complement-fixation is the preferred test.

Because of the serological relationships between R. rickettsii var pijperi and R. akari, only clinical findings may distinguish between South African tick-bite fever and rickettsial pox.

Rickettsia sibirinicus (Central Siberian tick typhus— Eastern Siberian tick typhus)

Agglutinins for Proteus OX 19 are present in both CS and ES tick typhus.

In ES tick typhus, agglutinins for OX 2 and OX K, at low titers, may be present.

The complement-fixation is the preferred test.

(c) Mite-borne rickettsial infections.

Rickettsia akari (Rickettsial pox)

Agglutination for the three types of Proteus is negative. For Proteus OX 19, however, it can be positive at low titers.

Rickettsia tsutsugamushi (Scrub typhus)

Only agglutinins for Proteus OX K appear. At high titers, over $\frac{1}{160}$, they are considered significant for the diagnosis of the disease. Low and negative titers, however, have been observed in ascertained R. tsutsugamushi infections. The complement-fixation test is more specific, but, in at least 50 per cent of the cases, C-F antibodies appear late or do not appear at all during the course of the disease.

(d) Rickettsial infections not necessarily borne by arthropods.

Rickettsia (Coxiella) burneti (Q fever)

Agglutination for the three strains of Proteus is constantly negative.

Agglutinins for R. burneti appear during the first week for 50 per cent of the cases, and in the second week for 90 per cent of the rest.

The titers may reach very high values.

The complement-fixation test, using antigens prepared with Henzerling (Italy) and Nine Mile (USA) strains is very reliable for diagnosis.

C-F antibodies appear somewhat later than the agglutinating ones. They may reach titers over $\frac{1}{1,000}$.

TESTS OF CHOICE IN RICKETTSIAL INFECTIONS DIAGNOSTIX

		SEROLOGIC TESTS			
		Agglutination			Complement-fixation
Etiologic Agent	*Disease*	*Proteus* OX 2	OX 19	OX K	
R. prowazeki	Epidemic typhus	+	++	0	+
	Brill's disease	+	++ irregular	0	+
R. mooseri	Murine typhus	0	++	0	+
R. quintana	Trench fever	0	0	0	+
R. rickettsi	American sp fever	++	++	0	+
R. brasiliensis	Sao Paulo typhus	+	+	+§	+
R. conori	Fiévre bouttoneuse	++	++	±	+
R. rickettsi var pijperi	S Afr tick bite fever	++	++	±	+
R. sibirinicus	Central and Eastern	0	++	0	+
R. australis	Siberian tick typhus	±	++	±	+
	North Queensland tick typhus	+	++	0	+
R. tsutsugamushi	Scrub typhus	0	0	++	+
R. akari	Rickettsial pox	0	0 occasionally low positivity	0	+
R. burneti	Q fever	0	0	0	+

§ A positive agglutination for Proteus OX L strain is observed.

12. PREPARATION OF RICKETTSIAL ANTIGENS FOR COMPLEMENT-FIXATION (C-F) TEST

Several methods have been devised to prepare rickettsial antigens. In the following paragraphs some of the basic steps will be described; it is, however, advisable to check current literature for the most suitable techniques.

Type specific washed antigens[24]

Incubate fertile hen eggs from six to eight days.

Inoculate a suspension of rickettsiae into the yolk sac; the suspension should be concentrated enough to kill the 5 to 10 per cent embryos after about four days.

On this day, remove eggs from incubator and keep at room temperature.[4]

On the seventh day after inoculation, harvest and weigh the yolk sacs.

Add half a volume of sterile ps.

Shake in a glass container with glass beads (a Waring blendor can be used) to grind the yolk sacs.

Suspend the material in sterile ps (pH 7.2) to a 20 per cent concentration of the original yolk sacs weight.

Add formaldehyde (40 per cent) to a concentration of 0.5 per cent.

Store the suspension at 5° C for seven days.

Centrifuge at 1,000 rpm for 10 min.

Draw off the mid-zone suspension and centrifuge at 4,500 rpm for 1 hr in angle-head centrifuge at a temperature of at least 4° C.

Discard the supernatant and swab carefully to remove any yolk sac stuck to the insides of the tubes.

Stir the sediment with a glass rod while adding, drop by drop, a 0.1 per cent formolized ps solution; accelerate the pouring of the diluent gradually, until the volume is equal to the original 20 per cent suspension.

Store for about 12 hr at 4° C.

Add an equal volume of a mixture of 90 per cent diethyl ether and 10 per cent ethyl alcohol and shake; a small volume of saline will quicken the separation of the mixture into three layers: the upper one containing excess of ether; the middle, tissue fragments and yolk particles, and the lower, aqueous, rickettsial and cell fragments.

The aqueous suspension is then extracted with ½ volume of the same ether-alcohol mixture.

Remove the excess ether with a suction pump.

Centrifuge the suspension at 4,500 rpm for 1 hr at 4° C.

Discard the supernatant and swab the tubes to remove fat.

Resuspend the sediment in a volume of ps equal to ⅒ of the original 20 per cent suspension.

Shake the suspension with washed, sterile Celite, using ¼₀ gm of the original tissue weight.

Centrifuge in angle head at 1,000 rpm for 30 min at 4° C.

Draw off the supernatant and centrifuge again at 4,500 rpm for 30 min at 4° C.

Suspend the sediment in ps to a volume equal to ¹⁄₁₀₀ of the original 20 per cent suspension.

Add formaldehyde to a concentration of 0.02 per cent.

Add Merthiolate to a concentration of ¹⁄₁₀,₀₀₀.

Store at 4° C.

Group specific soluble antigens[33]

Incubate and inoculate, as previously described, fertile hen eggs.

Harvest and weigh infected yolk sacs.

Squeeze out yolk from the bulk of yolk sacs.

Grind, as indicated above, with a little volume of sterile distilled H_2O.

Store at −20° C.

After a period of days or months, thaw and extract in 10 volumes of a mixture of 90 per cent diethyl ether and 10 per cent alcohol, shaking thoroughly, at 4° C for 1 hr.

Discard the ether and wash the tissue mass with the same ether-alcohol mixture until no more yellowish material dissolves.

Add ± 1.0 ml of sterile distilled H_2O for each gram of the original yolk sacs tissue and shake.

Remove the excess of ether with a vacuum pump.

Store at 4° C for about 12 hr.

Centrifuge the supernatant at 13,000 rpm for 30 min.
Add Merthiolate to a concentration of $\frac{1}{10,000}$ to the supernatant.
Store at $-20°$ C in order that the antigens may remain stable
for long periods—at $4°$ C for some months.

BIBLIOGRAPHY

1. BUGIARDINI, G.: *Arcisped S Anna Ferrara, 16*:541, 1963.
2. BUSBY, D. W. G., HOUSE, W., and McDONALD, J. R.: *Virological Technique*, First Edition, London, J. and A. Churchill, Ed., 1964, p. 143.
3. COMMISSION ON ACUTE RESPIRATORY DISEASES: *Amer J Med Sci, 208*:742, 1944.
4. COX, H. R.: *Ann N Y Acad Sci, 55*:326, 1952.
5. DULBECCO, R., and VOGT, M.: *J Exp Med, 99*:167, 1954.
6. FINLAND, M., and BARNES, M. W.: *Amer J Med Sci, 221*:152, 1951.
7. GIUNCHI, G., and SCURO, L. A.: In, INTROZZI, P., *Trattato Italiano di Medicina Interna, Part IV, Malattie Infettive e Parassitarie*, Roma, Abruzzini Ed., 1961, Vol. 2, p. 1,193.
8. HORSFALL, F. L., JR.: *Ann Intern Med, 27*:275, 1947.
9. HOYT, R. E., and MORRISON, L. M.: *Proc Soc Exp Biol Med, 93*: 547, 1956.
10. LENNETTE, E. H.: In, RIVERS, T. M., and HORSFALL, F. L.: *Viral and Rickettsial Infections of Man*, Third Edition, Philadelphia-Montreal, Lippincott Co., 1959, p. 234.
11. MELNICK, J. L.: In, *Diagnostic Procedures for Virus and Rickettsial Diseases*, Second Edition, New York City, Publication Office, American Public Health Assn., 1956, p. 128.
12. MELNICK, J. L., and OPTEN, E. M.: *Bull WHO, 14*:129, 1956.
13. MORRISON, L. M., and HOYT, R. E.: *J Lab Clin Med, 49*:774, 1957.
14. PAUL, J. R., and BUNNEL, W. W.: *Amer J Med Sci, 183*:90, 1932.
15. PAUL, J. R., and MELNICK, J. L.: In, *Diagnostic Procedures for Virus and Rickettsial Diseases*, Second Ed., New York City, Publication Office, American Public Health Assn., 1956, p. 73.
16. PAUL, J. R., and MELNICK, J. L.: *Ibid.*, p. 82.
17. PENSO, G., and BALDUCCI, D.: In, *Le Colture di Tessuti nella Ricerca Biologica*, First Ed., Roma, Il Pensiero Scientifico Ed., 1962, p. 225.
18. PENSO, G., and BALDUCCI, D.: *Ibid.*, p. 226.
19. PENSO, G., and BALDUCCI, D.: *Ibid.*, p. 228.
20. PENSO, G., and BALDUCCI, D.: *Ibid.*, p. 232.

21. PENSO, G., and BALDUCCI, D.: *Ibid.*, p. 235.
22. PENSO, G., and BALDUCCI, D.: *Ibid.*, p. 236.
23. PENSO, G., and BALDUCCI, D.: *Ibid.*, p. 244.
24. PLOTZ, H., BENNETT, B. L., WERTMAN, K., SNYDER, M. J., and GAULD, R. L.: *Amer J Hyg, 47:*150, 1948.
25. SALK, J. E., YOUNGER, J. S., and WARD, E. N.: *Amer J Hyg, 60:* 214, 1954.
26. SCHAUB, I. G., and FOLEY, M. K.: In, *Diagnostic Bacteriology.* London, Henry Kimpton, 1952, p. 282.
27. SCHAUB, I. G., and FOLEY, M. K.: *Ibid.*, p. 285.
28. SCHAUB, I. G., and FOLEY, M. K.: *Ibid.*, p. 287.
29. SEVER, J. L., HUEBNER, R. J., CASTELLANO, G. A., and BELL, J. A.: *Amer Rev Resp Dis, 88:*343, 1963.
30. SVEDMYR, A., ENDERS, J. F., and HOLLOWAY, A.: *Proc Soc Exp Biol Med, 79:*296, 1952.
31. THOMAS, L., MIRICK, G. S., CURNEN, E. C., ZIEGLER, J. E., and HORSFALL, F. L., JR.: *Science, 98:*566, 1943.
32. THOMAS, L., MIRICK, G. S., CURNEN, E. C., ZIEGLER, J. E., and HORSFALL, F. L., JR.: *J Clin Invest, 24:*227, 1945.
33. TOPPING, N. H., and SHEPARD, C. C.: *Public Health Rep, 61:*701, 1946.

V

SEROLOGICAL DIAGNOSTIX IN HEMATOLOGY

1. ERYTHROCYTES

Blood groups [8, 25, 27, 35, 51]

Erythrocytes have two agglutinogens, A and B, to which correspond anti-A and anti-B agglutinins in the serum. The presence of one or two, or the absence of agglutinogens, originate the group classification A, B, AB and O of the ABO system.

Two of the three fundamental genotypes—I^A, I^B, I^O— define the four groups. While I^A and I^B may combine, I^O is recessive to the first two. [35]

The presence of an agglutinogen excludes, of course, the presence of the homologous agglutinin in the serum.

Although five subgroups of A antigen are known, only the first two, A_1 and A_2, are of practical importance. [27, 36, 40, 49]

Individuals are classified as "secretors" (S) or "nonsecretors" (s) depending on whether soluble specific ABO substances are present or not in the saliva and other secretions. [1, 26, 27, 48]

A, B, O grouping

Using a known serum:

(a) *Preparation of the serum*

Store sterilely drawn blood at 4° C for 10 hr in order to eliminate cold hemagglutinins, if present.

Separate serum from clot immediately after removing from refrigerator.

Heat in water bath at 56° C for 20 min.

(b) *Titration of the serum*

Anti-A serum is provided by B-group donors; anti-B serum by A-group, and anti-AB by O-group.

Anti-A serum is titrated against A, A₁, AB, A₁B erythrocytes by the agglutination test; similarly, anti-B serum is titrated against B erythrocytes.

The minimal titers, indicated by the Bethesda National Institute of Health are $\frac{1}{256}$, for anti-A serum against A erythrocytes; $\frac{1}{128}$ against A₁ and A₁B erythrocytes; $\frac{1}{64}$ against A₂B erythrocytes, and $\frac{1}{256}$ for anti-B serum against B erythrocytes.

(c) *Titration of the serum avidity*

Serum avidity is titrated on the basis of the time necessary for agglutination to begin and on the ability to form agglutinates of at least 1 mm² in size.

Wash erythrocytes of groups A₁, A₂, A₁B, A₂B, and B twice and resuspend the sediment after the second centrifugation at 500 rpm for 3 min in saline to a 10 per cent concentration.

Mix 0.10 ml of A₁ erythrocytes suspension with 0.05 ml of anti-A serum on a glass. Start a chronometer immediately and shake gently, watching for agglutination.

When the agglutination appears, mark the time in seconds.

Continue shaking until the end of the third minute and measure the agglutinates.

Repeat the same process with A₂, A₁B, A₂B erythrocytes, using anti-B serum with B erythrocytes.

A good standard of avidity for a serum is the ability to form, in less than 3 min, agglutinates of at least 1 mm²: agglutination should start within 15 sec for A antiserum challenged with A₁ erythrocytes; within 30 sec when challenged with A₂ and A₁B erythrocytes; within 45 sec when challenged with A₂B erythrocytes; within 15 sec for B antiserum challenged with B erythrocytes.

In order to complete the above described tests, the following controls should be prepared:

(1) A cross-agglutination test, for specificity of the serum;

(2) Incubation at different temperatures (4, 12, 37° C) of equal volumes of two-fold dilutions of sera, and 10 per cent suspensions of erythrocytes in saline for 10 hr for cold agglutinins;

(3) Control for sterility of serum and erythrocytes, and
(4) Control of haemoglobin, which should not exceed 25 mg
   per cent.

Sera can be stored at 4° C, after addition of Merthiolate to ⅕,₀₀₀
concentration.

(d) *Typing of erythrocytes*

Draw 2.0 ml of blood from the patient, using a syringe moistened
   with heparin.
Centrifuge at 1,000 rpm for 5 min.
Discard the plasma.
Add 9.0 ml of saline to the erythrocytes, shake gently and centri-
   fuge.
Repeat this procedure twice again.
Discard supernatant and add saline making a 2 per cent suspen-
   sion.
(If the test is performed on dishes, a 5 per cent suspension is
   used.)
Place one drop of anti-A, anti-B, and anti-AB sera into each of
   three serology tubes.
Put one drop of erythrocytes suspension into each tube.
Repeat the whole procedure with an erythrocytes suspension of
   known group (A₁, B, or O).
Keep at room temperature for 10 min, or at 37° C if the presence
   of cold agglutinins is suspected.
Centrifuge at 1,000 rpm for 30 sec.
Read for results.

Interpretation of the results

If no agglutination is observed, the erythrocytes belong to
the O-group. If agglutination with anti-B and anti-AB sera is
observed, the erythrocytes belong to the B-group. If agglutination with anti-A and anti-AB sera is observed, the erythrocytes
belong to the A-group. If agglutination with anti-A, anti-B, and
anti-AB sera is observed, the erythrocytes belong to the AB
group.

Using an unknown serum

The technique is the same as that described above, but the

erythrocytes belong to known groups and the serum is unknown.

For titration, sera should be diluted in saline from $\frac{1}{2}$ up to $\frac{1}{1,028}$.

Interpretation of the results

If A_1 erythrocytes are agglutinated, the serum belongs to a B-group patient. If B erythrocytes are agglutinated, the serum belongs to an A-group patient. If A and B are agglutinated, the serum belongs to an O-group patient. If no agglutination takes place, the serum belongs to an AB-group patient.

A "complete test" for blood transfusions is performed by challenging:

(a) the recipient's serum with the donor's erythrocytes, and vice versa;

(b) the donor's and the recipient's erythrocytes with known anti-A and anti-B sera, and

(c) the donor's and the recipient's sera with known A and B erythrocytes.

Note: The correct interpretation of the test may be affected by several factors, as hemolysis or delay in the reading of the results; by transfusions of O-blood in individuals belonging to groups A and B, and by bacterial contamination of sera or erythrocytes. Some difficulties can be encountered in testing newborn babies or A (A_2, A_3) subgroups.

Subgroups A_1, A_2, A_1B, A_2B determination

1°—Using an absorbed serum

Absorb equal volumes of B serum on A_2 washed erythrocytes, keeping the suspension at 37° C for 1 hr.

Centrifuge at 1,000 rpm and recuperate supernatant.

Repeat absorption three more times.

Place one drop of the absorbed B serum in each of three separate tubes.

Add a standard A_1, A_2, and erythrocytes suspension to be tested in first, second, and third tubes.

Interpretation of the results

A_1 erythrocytes will be agglutinated; A_2 erythrocytes will not be agglutinated; erythrocytes tested will agglutinate if A_1, but will not agglutinate if A_2.

2°—*Using anti-O serum*

Prepare three sets of two-fold dilutions in saline of an O-anti-serum from $\frac{1}{2}$ up to $\frac{1}{1,024}$.

Add equal volumes of 2 per cent suspensions of A_1, A_2, and of the erythrocytes to be tested to the three sets.

Store at 22° C for 1 hr.

Centrifuge at 1,000 rpm for 30 sec.

Read for results.

Interpretation of the results

Low titer ($\frac{1}{8}$) agglutinations are observed with A_1 erythrocytes; high titer ($\frac{1}{128}$) agglutinations are observed with A_2 erythrocytes.

A, B, O group specific substances determination [12]

Titrate known antisera.

Heat saliva (or other body secretions to be tested) at 100° C for 10 min.

Filtrate with filter paper.

Dilute $\frac{1}{10}$ in saline.

Dilute $\frac{1}{16}$ A, B, or H antiserum.

Mix equal volumes of saliva and serum dilutions.

Store at 22° C for 15 min.

Titrate the mixture.

Interpretation of the results

A decrease in the titer of the serum after absorption reveals the presence of group-specific substances.

Rh blood groups [4, 10, 28, 37, 47]

The Rh system antigens are six: C, D, E, c, d, e; while d is hypothetical, the other ones are known.

Some variants have been studied, namely: D^u, C^w, C^x, E^w, E^u, e^x. D^u variant, indicated as a weak one, is of great importance in transfusions because even though it reacts weakly or not at all with anti-D sera, thus causing the labeling of erythrocytes as Rh−, it has active antigenic properties.

Rh testing

Preparation of the sera

Sera from naturally or artificially immunized individuals are employed. These sera should have a titer of at least $\frac{1}{32}$ and sufficient avidity (see page 95) to agglutinate Rh+ erythrocytes in 60 sec.

Sera from isoimmunized mothers generally reach a peak at the end of the first week after delivery.

To increase the titer, immunized individuals may sometimes be injected intravenously with erythrocytes having only the requested antigen. If necessary, both males and females in menopause can be immunized.

Antigen D (Rh_o) determination [30, 39, 50]

1°—Agglutination Test in Saline

Place 0.20 ml of anti-D (Rh_o) serum, having a titer of at least $\frac{1}{64}$ and sufficient avidity, in three serology tubes.

Add to the first tube 0.10 ml of d (rh) erythrocytes 2 per cent suspension in saline.

Add to the second tube 0.10 ml of D (Rh_o) erythrocytes 2 per cent suspension in saline.

Add to the third tube 0.10 ml of a 2 per cent suspension of the erythrocytes to be tested.

Shake well and incubate at 37° C for 1 hr.

Centrifuge at 1,000 rpm for 1 min.

Read for results.

2°—Agglutination Test by the "Albumin Method" with Sera Containing Incomplete Antibodies [24]

This test can be performed either in serology tubes or on dishes.

Place 0.10 ml of anti-D (Rh_o) test serum having a titer of at least $\frac{1}{64}$ and sufficient avidity into three serology tubes.

Add to the first tube 0.10 ml of a 2 per cent suspension of D (Rh$_o$) erythrocytes in 20 per cent bovine albumin.

Add to the second tube 0.10 ml of a 2 per cent suspension of d (rh) erythrocytes in 20 per cent bovine albumin.

Add to the third tube 0.10 ml of a 2 per cent suspension of the erythrocytes to be tested in 20 per cent bovine albumin (or in homologous serum or plasma).

Incubate at 37° C for 1 hr.

Centrifuge at 1,000 rpm for 1 min.

Read for results.

When dishes are used, slight differences in the technique are found.

Interpretation of the results

If agglutination is observed in tubes containing D and unknown erythrocytes, while the test is negative in the tube containing d erythrocytes, the blood examined is D type.

Several causes may alterate the results: low concentration of erythrocytes; excess of antiserum; delay in testing the blood, and agglutination test in saline when incomplete antibodies are present. The presence of D^u variants may also cause error in the interpretation of the results, due to its weakness in reacting with anti-D sera. When the presence of a D^u variant is suspected, it is necessary to perform a Moreschi-Coombs indirect test.

Moreschi-Coombs Indirect Test [31, 38]

Technique of the test

Place one drop of erythrocytes suspended in saline to 20 per cent concentration into a serology tube.

Add two drops of anti-D (Rh$_o$) serum, containing incomplete antibodies and having good avidity and an agglutination titer of at least 1/64.

Incubate at 37° C for 1 hr.

Wash erythrocytes four times and resuspend in saline at a 5 per cent concentration.

Mix one drop of erythrocytes suspension with one drop of anti-human gamma globulins serum into a cell slide.

Keep at 37° C for 10 to 15 min.

Read for results.

Interpretation of the test

If erythrocytes agglutinate, the blood belongs to the D^u type ($Rh_o{}^u$).

Note: Other antigens of the Rh system are studied using homologous antisera and employing the same technique.

M, N, S blood groups[9, 29]

M and N antigens are present in the erythrocytes and depend on the presence of two alleles L^M and L^N. Genotypes are $L^M L^M$, $L^N L^N$, $L^M L^N$ and the phenotypes are M, N, MN.

Anti-M and -N agglutinins are very rare.

As for the ABO system, weak variants M_2 and N_2 are seldom observed. In the MN system, the antigen S has been included together with its reciprocal s because the corresponding genes are placed in very close "loci" so that the two pairs are closely linked in inheritance.

MN and Ss types determination[13]

Preparation of the anti-M and -N sera

Anti-M and -N sera are obtained through the immunization of rabbits with M and N antigens.

Inject rabbits weighing ± 3 kg with 0.5 to 1.0 ml of erythrocytes of group O, type M or N, washed six times and suspended to 5 per cent concentration in saline, intravenously for five days.

Let the animals rest for seven days.

Inject subcutaneously, the first day after rest, with 0.5 to 1.0 ml of erythrocytes suspension, and intravenously the next day and every other day for a total of five intravenous injections.

Let the animals rest for one week.

Repeat the subcutaneous and intravenous series of injections.

Test for antibodies titer, and when a level of $\frac{1}{512}$ is reached bleed the animals and, after separation of serum at 37° C, inactivate at 56° C for 30 min.

Absorb aspecific and heterophil antibodies at 22° C for 1 hr on A_1 BM or A_1 BN erythrocytes previously washed in saline.

Preparation of the anti-S sera

Anti-S sera are uncommon and are obtained from human beings who have become immunized through repeated blood transfusions or pregnancy.

Determination of the M-N types

Set two rows of four serology tubes each.

Place one drop of anti-M serum into each tube of the first row.

Place one drop of anti-N serum into each tube of the second row.

Add to the four tubes of the first and second row one drop of a fresh 2 per cent suspension of erythrocytes in saline, respectively belonging to the types M, N, MN and the ones to be tested.

Keep at room temperature for 1 hr.

Centrifuge at 1,000 rpm for 1 min.

Read microscopically and macroscopically for agglutination.

Interpretation of the results

The type of the tested blood corresponds to the type of the agglutinated control erythrocytes.

Determination of the S antigen

The test is carried in saline or in bovine albumin, depending on the presence of complete or incomplete antibodies. In both cases, the incubation temperature is 37° C.

The technique is similar to the one described for the D antigen (See page 99.)

P blood groups [14]

Anti-P sera are obtained from immunized rabbits. Antibodies are most active at low temperatures and sometimes behave as hemolytic antibodies.

Lewis blood groups [14]

The Lewis system antigens are two: Le^a and Le^b.

Using an anti-Le^a serum it is possible to label Le^{a+} and Le^{a-} individuals.

Using also anti- Le^b serum it is possible to distinguish, in adults, three phenotypes: Le$^{(a + b-)}$, Le$^{(a - b +)}$, Le$^{(a - b -)}$.

Anti-Le^a antibodies have been observed both of natural or immune origin; antibodies of the first type are more active at room temperature and the second type at 37° C.

Kell-Cellano blood groups [13]

Antigens K (Kell) and k (Cellano) are defined by two alleles, K being the dominant.

K behaves as a strong antigen but being very rare, the cases of isoimmunization are relatively few.

The indirect Moreschi-Coombs test is employed to reveal the presence of the K antigen; for this purpose erythrocytes sensitized with anti-Kell serum are used.

Duffy blood groups [13]

The two alleles, Fy^a and Fy^b, can combine, and three phenotypes are obtained: Fy^{a}Fy^a, Fy^{a}Fy^b, Fy^{b}Fy^b.

The indirect Moreschi-Coombs test is used to reveal these antigens and erythrocytes to be tested are sensitized with anti-Fy serum.

Kidd blood groups [14]

The two alleles, JK^a and JK^b, can combine, and three phenotypes are obtained: JK^{a}JK^a, JK^{a}JK^b, JK^{b}JK^b.

Antibodies anti-JK react in saline, but it is preferable to employ the indirect Moreschi-Coombs test.

Jay blood groups [14]

Of the two alleles, Tj^a and Tj^b, only the first is present in almost 100 per cent of human beings. Tj^b is extremely rare.

Interreaction Tests [2]

Before performing a blood transfusion, the following tests are made to challenge the donor's erythrocytes with the recipient's serum.

Tests can be carried out in saline for anti-A, anti-B, or other complete antibodies; the indirect Moreschi-Coombs test is used to reveal the presence of incomplete antibodies in the recipient's serum.

Test in Saline

Mix, in a serology tube, 0.20 ml of the recipient's serum and 0.20 ml of a 2 per cent suspension in saline of the donor's erythrocytes.

Keep at room temperature for 2 hr.

Read for results.

Interpretation of the results

Agglutination, when present, may be due to anti-A, -B, or -M antibodies. Cold agglutinins may play a role in the agglutination; in this case, the upper limit of the temperature is 30° C, and the transfusion can be performed.

Indirect Moreschi-Coombs Test

Mix 1 volume of a 2 per cent suspension in saline of the washed donor's erythrocytes, with 5 volumes of the recipient's serum.

Incubate at 37° C for 2 hr.

Wash three times and resuspend (5 per cent) in saline.

Prepare a serial two-fold dilution in saline ($\frac{1}{4}$ to $\frac{1}{256}$), of anti-human globulins and distribute into serology tubes 0.10 ml of each dilution.

Add to each tube 0.10 ml of erythrocytes suspension.

Centrifuge at 1,000 rpm for 1 min.

Read for results.

Anti-D (Rh_o) and anti-Kell antibodies react better at high dilutions; anti-Le^a antibodies react better at low dilutions.

Interpretation of the results

If the test is positive, no blood transfusion should be performed.

ABO Isoantibodies [41]

Tests for anti-A and anti-B immune agglutinins

The following two tests are based on some characteristics of

natural and immune agglutinins. In the first test, the natural iso-
antibodies are absorbed on their soluble A and B antigens, while
immune agglutinins are not.

In the second test, the greater sensitivity of natural antibodies
to heat is used to reveal the presence of immune agglutinins.

(a) Challenge the serum to be tested and group specific AB
substance, at varying volumes, until the serum is completely deprived of its agglutinating activity. Once the optimum for neutralization is defined:

> neutralize 0.50 ml of serum to be tested, and
> follow the next technique, starting from the third step.

(b) Add to 1 volume of serum to be tested an equal amount of
saline:

Incubate in water bath at 70° C for 10 min.

Prepare 2 per cent suspensions of A and B erythrocytes in saline.

Prepare 2 per cent suspensions of A and B erythrocytes in bovine
albumin, diluted to 20 per cent in saline or in human AB
group serum.

Prepare two sets of serial two-fold dilutions of the serum, in saline, to a titer of $\frac{1}{1,024}$ (take into account, in preparing the
dilutions, the previous dilutions of serum for neutralization
or in saline).

Distribute 0.10 ml of each dilution into separate serology tubes.

Prepare two more sets of serum dilutions, as above, in bovine
albumin 20 per cent, or in human AB-group serum.

Place 0.10 ml of A and B erythrocytes suspensions in saline into
the first and second set of serum dilutions in saline.

Place 0.10 ml of A and B erythrocytes suspensions in bovine albumin (or AB group serum) into the third and fourth set of
serum dilutions.

Incubate at room temperature for 1 hr.

Centrifuge at 1,000 rpm for 1 min.

Read for results.

Interpretation of the results

The two sets of dilutions in saline should be negative due to the destruction of natural agglutinins by heat or by neutralization by AB group-specific AB substance.

If agglutination is observed in the third of fourth sets of dilutions in bovine albumin, immune agglutinins are present, and depending on the type of agglutinated erythrocytes, they belong to the anti-A or -B type.

Note: Besides anti-A and -B agglutinins, anti-A hemolysin is also present. To detect it, an hemolysis test is performed.

These procedures are very useful for the research of dangerous blood donors.

Technique of the test

Heat the serum to be tested at 56° C for 30 min in water bath.
Add, to 0.10 ml of serum, 0.10 ml of guinea pig complement and
     0.05 ml of A_1-group erythrocytes 5 per cent suspension.
Incubate in water bath at 37° C for 20 min.
Read for results.

Interpretation of the results

Avoid any transfusion if hemolysis is observed.

Note: Anti-O and anti-H antibodies agglutinate erythrocytes of O, A_2, A_2B-groups when challenged in saline at 16° C. Agglutination tests are performed to demonstrate the presence of such antibodies.

To state the type of antibody, the serum to be tested, after titration, is challenged with saliva of a secretor belonging to O-group; a decrease of the serum agglutinating titer proves the presence of anti-H agglutinins.

Technique for the demonstration of complete antibodies active at various temperatures [42]

Prepare two-fold serial dilutions in saline of the serum to be tested ($\frac{1}{2}$ to $\frac{1}{1,024}$).
Distribute 0.10 ml of each dilution in three sets of tubes.
Wash three times and suspend to 2 per cent concentration in saline the O-group erythrocytes, which have the wanted antigens.

Add 0.10 ml of the erythrocytes suspension to all the tubes con-
taining the serum dilutions.
Shake well and incubate.
First set of tubes at 4° C;
Second set of tubes at 12 to 20° C, and
Third set of tubes at 37° C.
After 10 hr interrupt incubation.
Read *immediately* for agglutination.

At the same time as that described above, prepare a test according to the:

Technique for the demonstration of complete and incomplete antibodies, active at various temperatures, by the "albumin method"[15]

Prepare two-fold dilutions of the serum to be tested, in bovine
albumin 20 per cent or in AB-group serum ($\frac{1}{2}$ to $\frac{1}{2,048}$).
Distribute in three sets of tubes 0.10 ml of each dilution.
Proceed with erythrocytes as described above.
Shake well and incubate.
First set of tubes at 4° C;
Second set of tubes at 12 to 18° C, and
Third set of tubes at 37° C.
Centrifuge all tubes at 1,000 rpm for 1 min.
Read microscopically and macroscopically for agglutination.

Interpretation of the results

When agglutination is observed, depending on whether the
reaction occurs in both saline and bovine albumin or just in bovine albumin, the presence of complete or incomplete antibodies
will be demonstrated.

The temperature at which the reaction has happened gives
the characteristic of such antibodies.

Technique for the demonstration of incomplete antibodies by the "trypsinized erythrocytes method"

The use of erythrocytes treated with proteolytic enzymes has
proved very useful in detecting incomplete antibodies.

Trypsinization of the erythrocytes [32] *

Prepare a 1 per cent solution of crystallin trypsin in HCl 0.05N.
Store at 4° C up to one week.

When used, dilute ⅒ the trypsin solution in phosphate buffer
  solution (pbs)† at pH 7.7, obtaining a 0.1 per cent concentration of trypsin.

Add to 0.2 ml washed erythrocytes of O-group having the antigen
  homologous to the antibody to be demonstrated, 1.0 ml of
  the 0.1 per cent trypsin solution.

Incubate at 37° C for 1 hr.

Wash erythrocytes three times in pbs.

Technique of the test

Prepare a two-fold serial dilution of the serum to be tested in
  saline (½ to ¹⁄₅₁₂).

Place 0.20 ml of undiluted serum and of its dilutions into ten separate serology tubes.

Add to each tube 0.10 ml of trypsinized, washed erythrocytes.

Shake well and incubate at 37° C for 1 hr.

Shake well and incubate for 1 hr more.

Read for agglutination.

Interpretation of the results

An agglutination titer over ¼ of the trypsinized erythrocytes
states for the presence of incomplete antibodies.

Direct Moreschi-Coombs Test [32]

(A) Technique for the warm, incomplete antibodies

Wash three times and suspend to 5 per cent in saline erythrocytes
  to be tested.

Mix into a serology tube equal volumes of erythrocytes suspension and human-globulin antiserum.

---

* Papain can be used in the place of trypsin; in this case, a different method
is used in the treatment of erythrocytes.

† Na_2HPO_4 — 1.63 per cent 90.5 ml
  $NaH_2PO_4 \cdot 2H_2O$ 2.34 per cent 9.5 ml

Prepare a control tube containing equal volumes of erythrocytes
suspension and saline.
Centrifuge at 1,000 rpm for 2 min.
Read for agglutination and, if negative,
Incubate at 37° C for 30 min.
Read again for agglutination.

Interpretation of the results

The agglutination of erythrocytes demonstrates the presence
of warm, incomplete antibodies.

Note: The test can be performed on dishes, in place of test
tubes, with few changes to the described standard method.

(B) *Technique for the cold, incomplete antibodies* [43]

Store blood at 4° C for serum separation; if lack of complement
is suspected, it is useful to add 1 volume of fresh normal serum
before storage.
Break clot and wash erythrocytes with warm (38 to 40° C) saline
several times.
Suspend erythrocytes in saline to 5 per cent concentration.
Perform a direct Moreschi-Coombs test as described above.

Interpretation of the results

Agglutination demonstrates the presence of cold, incomplete
antibodies.

Indirect Moreschi-Coombs Test

This test is employed to reveal the presence of free incomplete
antibodies in the serum.

The difference from the direct test consists in the fact that
the reaction occurs in two separate phases: a first one in which
the serum antibodies adhere to the erythrocytes antigens, and a
second one in which the anti-human globulin antibodies combine
with the globulin antigen of the serum.

Technique of the test

Wash O-group erythrocytes having the wanted antigen several
times, and suspend in saline to 5 per cent concentration.

Mix equal volumes of erythrocytes suspension and serum to be tested.

Incubate at 37° C for 1 hr.

Wash erythrocytes several times and resuspend in saline (5 per cent).

Mix equal volumes of erythrocytes suspension and anti-human globulin serum.

Incubate at 37° C for 30 min.

Centrifuge at 1,000 rpm for 30 min.

Read for agglutination.

Interpretation of the results

Agglutination demonstrates the presence of incomplete antibodies.

Note: An excessive washing treatment of erythrocytes may separate the antibody from the cells, while an inadequate one may allow an inhibition of the antiglobulin serum even by traces of the homologous serum.

To ascertain the warm or cold characteristics of the antibodies demonstrated with the Moreschi-Coombs tests, the following technique is applied:

Prepare on a dish, a four-fold dilution of 4 per cent human gamma globulins beginning from ¼ and up to $\frac{1}{4,096}$.

Add an equal amount of anti-human globulin serum to each dilution.

Keep at room temperature for 5 min.

Add to each antiserum-gamma globulin dilution an equal volume of a 5 per cent suspension of the erythrocytes to be tested after several washings.

Prepare the following controls:

(a) erythrocytes of O-group sensitized with anti-D (Rh$_o$) serum suspended to a 5 per cent concentration in saline, and

(b) same erythrocytes, but sensitized with cold, incomplete antibodies.‡

---

‡ Mix erythrocytes washed in saline with a serum known to contain cold, incomplete antibodies. Store at 0° C for 2 hr. Wash erythrocytes in warm (38 to 40° C) saline.

Treat control erythrocytes as described above.

Keep the three sets of tubes at room temperature for about 20 min.

Read for agglutination.

Interpretation of the results

If no agglutination is observed, the antibodies on the erythrocytes are of the warm, complete type; these antibodies behave as gamma globulins and hence the anti-human globulin serum, being absorbed on gamma globulins, is deprived of this fraction and cannot act on the erythrocytes sensitized with warm incomplete antibodies.

On the contrary, if agglutination is observed the antibodies are of the cold, incomplete type; these antibodies do not behave as gamma globulins and hence the anti-human globulins serum, absorbed on gamma globulins though deprived of this fraction, acts on the erythrocytes sensitized with cold, incomplete antibodies.

Moreschi-Coombs Test for Blocking Antibodies [3]

Wash several times and suspend to 2 per cent concentration in saline erythrocytes from various Rh+ and Rh− bloods.

Place one drop of each suspension into as many serology tubes.

Add to each tube one drop of the serum to be tested.

Incubate the whole lot of tubes at 37° C for 1 hr.

Fill up with saline and shake well all the tubes.

Centrifuge all the tubes at 1,000 rpm for 1 min and discard the supernatant.

Repeat washing and centrifuging three more times.

Discard the last supernatant and resuspend cells in one drop of saline.

Add to each tube one drop of anti-human globulins serum and shake well.

Keep for 5 min at room temperature and then centrifuge at 500 rpm for 2 min.

Shake gently the tubes.

Read for results.

Interpretation of the results

Agglutination of erythrocytes, absent on ordinary anti-Rh antibodies test, indicates the presence of blocking antibodies for those particular Rh antigens.

Test for Warm and Cold, Acid-Sensible Hemolysins

Acidify serum to be tested using HCl N/3.5 to pH 6.8.§

Repeat such procedure with guinea pig complement (or fresh, known negative serum).

Prepare a two-fold serial dilution of the acidified serum, from ½ up to $\frac{1}{256}$, using as a diluent either the acidified guinea pig complement or the fresh serum.

Distribute 0.20 ml of each dilution into separate tubes.

Incubate all the tubes at 37° C (at 12° C for cold hemolysins) in water bath for 20 min.

Add 0.10 ml of a washed 10 per cent suspension in saline of O-group erythrocytes.

Incubate at 37° C for 2 hr.

|| Read for results.

Interpretation of the test

The presence of acid-sensible hemolysins is demonstrated by hemolysis of the system.

Test for Diphasic Hemolysins [44]

Draw blood with a syringe warmed at 37° C, and distribute to two serology tubes, A and B.

Incubate tube A at 37° C and tube B at 0° C for 30 min.

Transfer tube B to 37° C.

Incubate for 1 hr.

Read for results.

Interpretation of the results

If diphasic hemolysin is present, hemolysis is observed in tube B.

---

§ Erythrocytes can be pretreated with trypsin (see page 108) and acidification avoided. Controls should be prepared using normal sera.

|| The presence of an anticomplementary effect by the serum to be tested can be overcome, replacing it with fresh serum after contact with erythrocytes. If hemolysins are present, a quick hemolysis appears.

2. LEUKOCYTES

Test for Leukolysins [18, 19, 45]

In this test a per cent evaluation of leukolysis is obtained.

Technique of the test [21, 23]

Place 1.0 ml of leukocytes suspension ¶ into three separate ser-
ology tubes (a), (b), and (c).
Add 1.0 ml of the serum to be tested to tube (a),
    add 1.0 ml of normal serum to tube (b), and
    add 1.0 ml of Ringer-Locke solution ** to tube (c).
Incubate at 37° C for 1 hr.
Shake and read microscopically on a Bürker hemocytometer.

Interpretation of the results

The per cent of leukolysis is calculated with the difference in
number of leukocytes of (a), (b), and (c) suspensions.

Test for Leukoagglutinins [20]

Inactivate serum to be tested and a control normal serum at 56° C
    for 30 min.
Prepare two-fold serial dilutions of both sera, from ½ up to $\frac{1}{128}$,
    or over.
Distribute 0.10 ml of the dilutions in two sets of separate serology
    tubes.
Place 0.10 ml of saline into one tube for control of agglutination.
Add to all tubes 0.05 ml of leukocytes suspension. [21, 23]

¶ Defibrinate 30.0 ml of O-group blood by means of sterile glass beads on a
rotating shaker at 60 rot/min for 15 min.

Transfer 15.0 ml of defibrinated blood to a new sterile tube.
Add 3.0 ml of 3.5 per cent sterile solution of polyvinyl-pyrroliodone.
Incubate at 37° C for 30 min in an inclinate position.
Draw off gently the supernatant which contains ± 4,000 cells cubic milli-
    meter.
The leukocytes suspensions should be promptly used.

** NaCl   9.0 gm ⎫ dissolve in 500.0 ml distilled H_2O—add distilled H_2O
   Na_2CO_3 0.2 gm ⎬ to 1,000 ml.
   $CaCl_2$ 0.2 gm ⎭

Shake well and incubate at 36° C for 30 min.

Add one drop of 1 per cent acetic acid solution to all tubes and
shake well.

Immediately place one drop from each tube on glass slides.

Read for agglutination.

Interpretation of the results

Agglutination is considered as positive when clumping of
5 to 20 leukocytes is observed.

The titer is given by the highest dilution of serum in which
agglutination is observed.

Normal control serum and saline should not agglutinate leukocytes.

3. PLATELETS

The presence in sera of antibodies causing lysis or agglutination of platelets can be demonstrated by a number of tests. The
more commonly used in routine work will be described.

Lysis evaluation by platelets count [46]

Prepare a platelets suspension †† and distribute 1.0 ml of it into
three separate siliconed serology tubes.

Add to each tube 1.0 ml of serum to be tested, 1.0 ml of fresh
normal serum, and 1.0 ml of bps.

Make a platelet count for each suspension.

Stop tubes with rubber stoppers and incubate at 37° C for 3 hr.

Shake tubes gently and repeat platelet count.

Interpretation of the results

By the difference in number of platelets between the two

---

†† To prepare a platelets suspension: [22]

Add to 9.0 ml of group-O normal blood, 1.0 ml of a 5 per cent sequestrene
solution in NaCl 0.85 per cent.

Centrifuge at 3,000 rpm for 2 min.

Recuperate the supernatant plasma and centrifuge again at 1,000
rpm for 5 min.

The final suspension contains about 300,000 platelets cubic millimeter and
may be stored at 4° C for about 5 hr.

counts, a per cent value of thrombolytic activity of the tested serum is obtained.

Other methods are based on the medium clarification due to cells lysis, and on the morphologic modifications of cells.

Agglutination Test[22]

Inactivate serum to be tested by heating at 56° C for 30 min.

Place two drops of serum in several concavities of a multiple depression tray.

Add one drop of platelets suspension to each concavity containing serum (platelets suspensions from different normal individuals should be used for better control of the test).

A couple of normal, inactivated sera should be used as controls.

Place the tray on a platform-type rotator.

Operate at 110 rotations per min at room temperature, or at 4° C, for 20 min.

Read microscopically for results.

Interpretation of the results

The test is positive when 10 to 20 platelets are agglutinated together. The degree of positivity is indicated from 1 to 4+, depending on the size of agglutinates.

Direct Moreschi-Coombs Test for Incomplete Thrombo-Agglutinins[16, 22]

Prepare a two-fold dilution in physiologic saline (ps) of rabbit anti-human globulins, from $\frac{1}{2}$ to $\frac{1}{128}$.

Distribute two drops of each dilution in separate cells of a multiple depression glass tray.

Add one drop of platelets suspension to be tested (see page 114) containing about 500,000 cells cubic millimeter to each serum dilution.

Add one drop of platelets suspension to two drops of ps for auto-agglutination control.

Repeat the whole procedure on a normal platelets suspension for control of rabbit anti-human globulins serum.

Place the tray on a platform-type rotator.

Operate at 110 rpm for 5 min at room temperature.
Read microscopically for results.

Interpretation of the results

Agglutination of platelets tested indicates the presence of incomplete antibodies *in vivo*.

Controls should not agglutinate.

Indirect Moreschi-Coombs Test for Incomplete Thrombo-Agglutinins [17]

Prepare a platelets suspension (see page 114) from Normal O-group blood, containing about 200,000 cells cubic millimeter.

Inactivate serum to be tested and normal control sera at 56° C for 30 min.

Absorb 1.0 ml of each serum on 0.1 gm of barium sulphate at 37° C for 30 min.

Centrifuge sera at 3,000 rpm for 10 min and recuperate supernatant sera.

Mix 0.3 ml of each serum with 0.15 ml of platelets suspension (use silicon-treated tubes) and agitate on rotator in a sloping position at 4° C for 90 min.

Wash platelets twice in pbs ‡‡ at pH 7.6.

Add to the sedimented platelets 0.10 ml of rabbit anti-human globulins serum, diluted ¼.

Place tubes on rotator in a sloping position and agitate at room temperature for 30 min.

Read microscopically for agglutination.

Interpretation of the results

As described above.

BIBLIOGRAPHY

1. BOORMAN, K. E., and DODD, B. E.: *J Path Bact*, 55:329, 1943.
2. BOYD, W. C.: In, *Fundamentals of Immunology*. Third Ed., New York, Interscience Publishers, Inc., 1956, p. 644.
3. BOYD, W. C.: *Ibid.*, p. 651.

---

‡‡ Phosphate buffered solution:
PO_4HNa_2 9.4 per cent solution: 2 volumes.
Sequestrene 1 per cent solution in NaCl 0.85 per cent: 1 volume.

4. BROMAN, B.: *Acta Paediat, 31*:1, Suppl. 2, 1944.
5. COOMBS, R. R. A., GLEESON-WHITE, W. H., and HALL, J. G.: *Brit J Exp Path, 32*:195, 1951.
6. COOMBS, R. R. A., and MOURANT, A. E.: *J Path Bact, 59*:105, 1947.
7. COOMBS, R. R. A., MOURANT, A. E., and RACE, R. R.: *Brit J Exp Path, 26*:255, 1945.
8. DAUSSET, J.: In, *Immuno-Hematologie Biologique et Clinique.* Paris, Ed. Med. Flammarion, 1956, p. 21.
9. DAUSSET, J.: *Ibid.,* p. 50.
10. DAUSSET, J.: *Ibid.,* p. 121.
11. DAUSSET, J.: *Ibid.,* p. 385.
12. DAUSSET, J.: *Ibid.,* p. 397.
13. DAUSSET, J.: *Ibid.,* p. 401.
14. DAUSSET, J.: *Ibid.,* p. 406.
15. DAUSSET, J.: *Ibid.,* p. 430.
16. DAUSSET, J.: *Ibid.,* p. 568.
17. DAUSSET, J.: *Ibid.,* p. 570.
18. DAUSSET, J.: *Ibid.,* p. 602.
19. DAUSSET, J.: *Ibid.,* p. 673.
20. DAUSSET, J.: *Ibid.,* p. 675.
21. DAUSSET, J.: *Rev Franç Étud Clin Biol, 1*:241, 1956.
22. DAUSSET, J., and MALINVAUD, G.: *Le Sang, 25*:847, 1954.
23. DAUSSET, J., NENNA, A., and BRECY, H.: *Blood, 9*:696, 1954.
24. DIAMOND, L. K., and DENTON, R. L.: *J Lab Clin Med, 30*:821, 1945.
25. DUJARRIC DE LA RIVIÈRE, R., and KOSSOVITCH, N.: *Ann Inst Pasteur, 55*:331, 1935.
26. FORMAGGIO, T. G.: *Minerva Medicoleg, 71*:157, 1951.
27. GIUNCHI, G.: In, *Compendio di Immunoematologia.* Clinica Medica, Università di Roma, Napoli, G. D'Agostino Ed., 1954, p. 11.
28. GIUNCHI, G.: *Ibid.,* p. 91.
29. GIUNCHI, G.: *Ibid.,* p. 128.
30. HABERMANN, S., and HILL, J. M.: *Brit. Med J, 1*:851, 1952.
31. HILL, J. M., and HABERMANN, S.: *Amer J Clin Path, 24*:305, 1954.
32. INTROZZI, P.: In, *Trattato Italiano di Medicina Interna.* Tecniche e Diagnostica di Laboratorio, Roma, Abruzzini Ed., 1960, Vol 2, p. 888.
33. INTROZZI, P.: *Ibid.,* p. 889.
34. INTROZZI, P.: *Ibid.,* p. 890.
35. LANDSTEINER, K.: *Zbl Bakt, 27*:357, 1900.
36. LANDSTEINER, K., and LEVINE, K.: *J Immun, 18*:87, 1930.

118   *Serological Diagnostix*

37. LANDSTEINER, K., and WIENER, A. S.: *J Exp Med, 74*:309, 1941.
38. MORESCHI, C.: *Zbl Bakt, 46*:49, 1908.
39. MOURANT, A. E.: *Rev Hémat, 4*:111, 1949.
40. MOUREAU, P.: *Bull Acad Roy Med Belg, 8*:31, 1943.
41. NINNI, M., and BEDARIDA, G.: In, INTROZZI, P., *Trattato Italiano di Medicina Interna,* Tecniche e Diagnostica di Laboratorio, Roma, Abruzzini Ed., 1960, Vol. 2, p. 885.
42. NINNI, M., and BEDARIDA, G.: *Ibid.*, p. 887.
43. NINNI, M., and BEDARIDA, G.: *Ibid.*, p. 890.
44. NINNI, M., and BEDARIDA, G.: *Ibid.*, p. 893.
45. NINNI, M., and BEDARIDA, G.: *Ibid.*, p. 902.
46. NINNI, M., and BEDARIDA, G.: *Ibid.*, p. 919.
47. RACE, R. R., TAYLOR, G. L., BOORMAN, K. E., and DODD, B. E.: *Nature, 152*:563, 1943.
48. WIENER, A. S., and KOSOFKY, I.: *J Immun, 42*:381, 1941.
49. WIENER, A. S., and SILVERMAN, I. J.: *Amer J Clin Path, 11*:45, 1941.
50. WIENER, A. S., and SONN, E. B.: *Ann NY Acad Sci, 46*:969, 1946.
51. WIENER, A. S., and WEXLER, L. B.: *Bact Rev, 16*:69, 1952.

INDEX